THE HEART HEALTHY COOKBOOK FOR BEGINNERS

Discover Delicious and Nutritious Low-Fat Recipes to Support a Strong Heart. Includes a 30-Day Meal Plan, and Expert Guidance for Optimal Health!

TABLE OF CONTENTS

INTRODUCTION 8
WHAT IS HEART DISEASE? 10
   Causes of Heart Disease 11
   How Heart Disease is Treated 13
   Benefits of the Heart-Healthy Eating Pattern.. 14
   Tips and Tricks for Following a Healthy Eating Pattern 15
   What to Eat and What to Avoid.. 18
BREAKFAST RECIPES 21
      BANANA OAT PANCAKES 22
      SPINACH AND MUSHROOM EGG WHITE SCRAMBLE 22
      OVERNIGHT CHIA PUDDING.. 23
      AVOCADO AND TOMATO TOAST 23
      APPLE CINNAMON QUINOA BREAKFAST BOWL 24
      VEGGIE AND EGG BREAKFAST BURRITO 24
      GREEK YOGURT AND BERRY PARFAIT 25
      PEANUT BUTTER AND BANANA SMOOTHIE............................... 25
      VEGETABLE OMELET.. 26
      BERRY OATMEAL... 26
      TROPICAL GREEN SMOOTHIE 27
      COTTAGE CHEESE AND FRUIT BOWL... 27
      MULTIGRAIN WAFFLES WITH FRUIT 28
      ALMOND BUTTER AND APPLE RICE CAKES................................ 28
      SPINACH, TOMATO, AND MOZZARELLA FRITTATA 28
      SMOKED SALMON AND AVOCADO RICE CAKE........................... 29
      TURKEY SAUSAGE AND VEGGIE SCRAMBLE 29
      CHIA PUDDING WITH FRUIT..30
      GREEK YOGURT WITH GRANOLA AND BERRIES 30
      AVOCADO AND EGG TOAST 31
      PINEAPPLE, BANANA, AND SPINACH SMOOTHIE 31

- QUINOA AND BERRY BREAKFAST BOWL 32
- GREEN DETOX SMOOTHIE 32
- VEGGIE AND HUMMUS WRAP 32
- COTTAGE CHEESE AND FRUIT BOWL 33

.... 34

SNACK RECIPES 34
- SPICY ROASTED CHICKPEAS 35
- GREEK YOGURT RANCH DIP WITH VEGGIES 35
- APPLE SLICES WITH ALMOND BUTTER 35
- MINI CAPRESE SKEWERS 36
- CELERY STICKS WITH CREAM CHEESE AND EVERYTHING BAGEL SEASONING 36
- AVOCADO-STUFFED CHERRY TOMATOES 36
- CUCUMBER SLICES WITH HUMMUS 37
- ANTS ON A LOG 37
- EASY EDAMAME 37
- PEANUT BUTTER AND CHOCOLATE RICE CAKES 37
- SPINACH AND ARTICHOKE DIP 38
- FRUIT KABOBS WITH HONEY-YOGURT DRIP 38
- SLICED TURKEY AND CHEESE ROLL-UPS 38
- POPCORN WITH NUTRITIONAL YEAST 39
- BELL PEPPER NACHOS 39
- VEGGIE PINWHEELS 40
- FROZEN YOGURT BARK 40
- CHOCOLATE BANANA BITES 40
- SMOKED SALMON AND CREAM CHEESE CUCUMBER BITES 41
- CHEESE AND CRACKERS 41

MEAT RECIPES 42
- TURKEY MEATBALLS 43
- PORK TENDERLOIN WITH BALSAMIC GLAZE 43
- BEEF STIR-FRY WITH BROCCOLI 44
- BAKED CHICKEN FAJITA STUFFED PEPPERS 44
- GREEK-STYLE GRILLED CHICKEN 45

BALSAMIC-GLAZED PORK CHOPS 46
BEEF AND VEGETABLE STIR-FRY 46
SLOW COOKER BEEF STEW 47
SHEET PAN SAUSAGE AND VEGETABLES 47
CHICKEN AND RICE STUFFED BELL PEPPERS 48
SPAGHETTI SQUASH BOLOGNESE 49
GARLIC HERB PORK TENDERLOIN 49
CHICKEN AND BROCCOLI STIR-FRY 50
TURKEY MEATBALL SUBS 51
GRILLED PORTOBELLO MUSHROOM BURGERS 51
GREEK CHICKEN PITA POCKETS 52
PHILLY CHEESESTEAK STUFFED PEPPERS 53
BBQ-PULLED CHICKEN SANDWICHES 53
BEEF AND VEGETABLE-STIR FRY 54
BALSAMIC GLAZED CHICKEN 55
SAUSAGE, PEPPERS, AND ONIONS SKILLETS 56
ROSEMARY LEMON PORK CHOPS 56
MOROCCAN-SPICED BEEF STEW 57
SPINACH AND FETA STUFFED CHICKEN BREASTS 58
ASIAN TURKEY LETTUCE WRAPS 58

SEAFOODS RECIPE 60
LEMON GARLIC BAKED COD 61
SHRIMP AND VEGGIE STIR-FRY 61
PAN-SEARED SCALLOPS WITH GARLIC SPINACH 62
SALMON WITH DILL YOGURT SAUCE 62
CRAB CAKES WITH LEMON AIOLI 63
ONE-PAN SHRIMP AND ASPARAGUS 64
BAKED TILAPIA WITH MEDITERRANEAN SALSA 64
EASY CLAM SPAGHETTI 65
SEARED AHI TUNA WITH MANGO SALSA 65
SEAFOOD PAELLA 66
BAKED COD WITH CHERRY TOMATOES AND OLIVES 66
GARLIC BUTTER SCALLOPS 67

- LEMON HERB BAKED SALMON 68
- SPICY CAJUN SHRIMP SKILLET 68
- MISO-GLAZED SALMON 69
- SHRIMP SCAMPI 69
- SHRIMP AND SPINACH STUFFED PORTOBELLO MUSHROOMS 71
- TERIYAKI GLAZED SALMOND 71
- SEAFOOD-STUFFED BELL PEPPERS 72
- LEMON GARLIC SHRIMP AND ASPARAGUS 73
- PESTO BAKED SCALLOPS 73
- TILAPIA WITH LEMON CAPER SAUCE 74
- SPICY ORANGE GLAZED SHRIMP 74
- POACHED COD WITH TOMATO SALSA 75
- LOBSTER AND CORN CHOWDER 75

SOUPS RECIPES 77
- TOMATO BASIL SOUP 78
- SPINACH AND WHITE BEAN SOUP 78
- SPICED LENTIL SOUP 79
- MUSHROOM BARLEY SOUP 79
- BUTTERNUT SQUASH AND APPLE SOUP 80
- CHICKEN AND VEGETABLE SOUP 80
- CREAMY CAULIFLOWER SOUP 81
- MINESTRONE SOUP 82
- POTATO LEEK SOUP 82
- ROASTED RED PEPPER AND TOMATO SOUP 83
- HEARTY VEGETABLE AND BARLEY SOUP 83
- WHITE BEAN AND KALE SOUP 84
- CREAMY MUSHROOM SOUP 84
- SPICED RED LENTIL SOUP 85
- ZUCCHINI AND CORN CHOWDER 85
- MISO VEGETABLE SOUP 86
- CABBAGE AND POTATO SOUP 87
- PEA AND MINT SOUP 87
- POTATO AND LEEK SOUP 88

- CARROT AND GINGER SOUP 88
- 90

VEGETABLE RECIPES 90
- GARLIC-ROASTED BRUSSELS SPROUTS 91
- CAULIFLOWER FRIED RICE 91
- BALSAMIC GLAZED CARROTS 91
- CURRIED CHICKPEA AND SPINACH 92
- STUFFED BELL PEPPERS 92
- SWEET POTATO AND BLACK BEAN HASH 93
- LEMON-GARLIC GEREN BEANS 93
- SPICY ROASTED CAULIFLOWER 94
- STOVETOP RATATOUILLE 94
- PARMESAN ROASTED BROCCOLI 95
- GREEN BEANS ALMONDINE 95
- GARLIC MASHED CAULIFLOWER 96
- SAUTÉED SPINACH WITH GARLIC 96
- SWEET AND SOUR RED CABBAGE 97
- OVEN-ROASTED ROOT VEGETABLE 97
- EGGPLANT PARMESAN STACKS 98
- CREAMY POLENTA WITH ROASTED VEGETABLES 98
- STUFFED PORTOBELLO MUSHROOMS 99
- ZUCCHINI FRITTERS 100
- CHICKPEA AND VEGETABLE CURRY 100

DESSERT RECIPES 102
- EASY FRUIT SALAD 103
- CHOCOLATE AVOCADO MOUSSE 103
- BAKED CINNAMON APPLE SLICES 103
- COCONUT RICE PUDDING 104
- RASPBERRY LEMON SORBET 104
- CHOCOLATE-DIPPED BANANA BITES 105
- MINI FRUIT TARTS 106
- LEMON BLUEBERRY CHIA PUDDING 106
- STRAWBERRY BANANA SMOOTHIE BOWL 107

- MANGO COCONUT POPSICLES 107
- PINEAPPLE COCONUT MACAROONS 108
- ALMOND APRICOT BITES 108
- BAKED CINNAMON APPLES 108
- FRUIT KABOBS WITH HONEY YOGURT DIP 109
- DARK CHOCOLATE BARK WITH DRIED FRUIT AND NUTS 109

COVERSION TABLES 112
- VOLUME CONVERSION 112
- WEIGHT CONVERSION 112
- LENGTH COVERSION 112
- TEMPERATURE CONVERSION 112

30 DAY MEAL PLAN 113

CONCLUSION **119**

INDEX **121**

INTRODUCTION

Maintaining a healthy lifestyle is becoming increasingly challenging in our fast-paced world. The ubiquity of heart disease, which is one of the primary reasons for mortality across the world, serves as evidence to support this assertion. The positive news, nevertheless, is that various types of heart disease can be averted or regulated via healthy dietary habits and lifestyle selections.

This comprehensive cookbook was meticulously crafted for individuals who aspire to lead a heart-healthy lifestyle, making it an ideal resource for those who are commencing their journey. Changing your eating habits can be scary, which is why this book is here to help you every step of the way. It discusses the significance of maintaining long-term heart health and provides a variety of recipes that you and your family can enjoy for decades.

This cookbook aims to debunk the myth that heart-healthy eating is synonymous with bland, tasteless food. On the contrary, the recipes featured in this book showcase the natural flavors and richness of whole, nutrient-dense ingredients. You'll discover that heart-healthy cuisine can be just as tasty, if not more so, than the standard diet by using herbs, spices, and other natural flavor enhancers.

This cookbook not only emphasizes the nutritional components of a heart-healthy diet but also stresses the value of moderation and balance. By incorporating a variety of foods and ingredients, you'll ensure that your body receives all the necessary nutrients to thrive. You'll learn to listen to your body and to make mindful choices about the foods you consume, ultimately leading to a healthier, more fulfilling life.

As you embark on your heart-healthy journey, you'll also gain invaluable knowledge about nutrition's vital role in preventing and managing heart disease. This cookbook provides a solid foundation for understanding how certain ingredients and cooking techniques can promote optimal heart health. You'll become more informed about the benefits of various food groups and how to incorporate them into your diet in a balanced and delicious manner.

In addition to physical health benefits, adopting a heart-healthy lifestyle can significantly impact your emotional and mental well-being. By prioritizing self-care and investing in your health, you'll likely experience increased energy levels, improved mood, and a heightened sense of accomplishment. This cookbook is a collection of recipes and an empowering tool to help you take control of your health and improve your overall quality of life.

As you explore the pages of this cookbook, you'll realize that a heart-healthy diet is not a temporary fix but a lifelong commitment to wellness. And with the flavorful, low-sodium, and low-fat recipes at your fingertips, you'll be well-equipped to make this commitment both enjoyable and sustainable. Here's to a lifetime of heart-healthy living!

WHAT IS HEART DISEASE?

Cardiovascular disease, commonly known as heart disease, refers to a set of health conditions that impact the function and appearance of the heart and blood vessels. These ailments can impede the heart's capacity to effectively circulate blood, furnish the body's tissues with oxygen and nutrients, and sustain a steady heartbeat. People often use the terms "heart disease" and "cardiovascular disease" interchangeably, even though "heart disease" refers only to conditions that affect the heart, and "cardiovascular disease" includes conditions that affect both the heart and blood vessels.

Outlined below are some of the most prevalent types of heart disease:

1. Coronary Artery Disease (CAD)

This is the most prevalent form of heart disease. This occurs when plaque, a buildup of fatty deposits, accumulates within the arteries that supply blood to the heart muscle, leading to constriction or blockage of these vessels. Diminished blood circulation can result in chest discomfort (angina), breathing difficulties, and other indications. A plaque rupture can lead to a blood clot that obstructs the artery, causing a heart attack.

2. Heart Failure

Also referred to as congestive heart failure, this disorder emerges when the heart is unable to pump a sufficient amount of blood to meet the body's requisites. Heart failure can arise from various elements, including CAD, elevated blood pressure, or harm to the heart muscle from a prior heart attack.

3. Arrhythmias

These irregular heart rhythms may arise from anomalies in the heart's electrical system. Heart arrhythmias can cause the heart to beat excessively fast, too slow, or in an otherwise irregular pattern. Atrial fibrillation, bradycardia, and tachycardia are all common types of arrhythmias.

4. Heart Valve Disease

When one or more of the heart's valves malfunction, it can disrupt blood flow within the heart, leading to a condition called valvular heart disease. Valve problems can be congenital (present at birth) or develop over time due to aging, infections, or other factors.

5. Cardiomyopathy

This pertains to disorders of the heart muscle that can enfeeble the heart and impede its ability to effectively circulate blood. Several types of cardiomyopathy include dilated, hypertrophic, and restrictive cardiomyopathy.

6. Congenital Heart Defects

These are problems with the heart that are already there at birth, like a hole in the heart, bad valves, or problems with the chambers of the heart. Some congenital heart defects are mild and may not cause symptoms, while others can be more severe and require treatment early in life.

7. Pericardial Disease

This encompasses predicaments with the pericardium, the thin sac that encloses and safeguards the heart. Conditions like pericarditis (inflammation of the pericardium), pericardial effusion (fluid buildup around the heart), and constrictive pericarditis (thickening and scarring of the pericardium) can affect how the heart works and cause symptoms like chest pain and shortness of breath.

Causes of Heart Disease

There are many things that can lead to heart disease.

Some of the primary causes include:

1. High Blood Pressure (hypertension)

Persistently elevated blood pressure can impair the blood vessels and the heart, augmenting the likelihood of heart disease.

2. High Cholesterol

Elevated levels of low-density lipoprotein (LDL) cholesterol, also known as "bad" cholesterol, can lead to plaque buildup in the arteries, contributing to the development of CAD.

3. Smoking

Smoking has detrimental effects on blood vessels and can lead to atherosclerosis, a condition characterized by the constriction of the arteries. This makes heart disease more likely.

4. Obesity

Excessive weight places added strain on the heart and can worsen pre-existing conditions such as high blood pressure, high cholesterol, and diabetes, ultimately augmenting the chance of developing heart disease.

5. Diabetes

When blood sugar levels are too high, blood vessels and nerves can get hurt. This makes heart disease more likely.

6. Sedentary lifestyle

Physical inactivity can be a contributing factor to obesity, elevated blood pressure, and high cholesterol, thereby amplifying the hazard of heart disease.

7. Genetics and family history

A family history of heart disease can increase an individual's risk due to genetic factors and shared lifestyle habits.

Symptoms of Heart Disease

Manifestations of heart disease may differ contingent on the precise condition; nevertheless, some shared symptoms may encompass the following:

- Chest pain or discomfort (angina)
- Shortness of breath
- Dizziness or lightheadedness
- Fatigue
- Irregular heartbeat (arrhythmia)
- Swelling in the extremities (edema)
- Rapid weight gain
- Nausea or lack of appetite
- Persistent cough or wheezing

How Heart Disease is Treated

Treatment options for heart disease depend on the severity and underlying cause of the condition.

Some common treatment approaches include:

1. Medications

Various medications can be used to treat heart diseases, such as blood pressure-lowering drugs, cholesterol-lowering drugs (statins), antiplatelet medications, anticoagulants, and medications to control heart rate and rhythm.

2. Lifestyle Changes

Embracing a heart-healthy way of life is crucial in preventing and regulating heart disease. This includes consuming a balanced diet, engaging in regular exercise, maintaining a healthy weight, giving up smoking, and managing stress.

3. Medical Procedures

In certain instances, medical procedures may be necessary to address heart disease. These can include angioplasty (a procedure to open blocked arteries), stenting (inserting a small mesh tube to keep an artery open), and bypass surgery (surgically creating a new route for blood flow around a blocked artery).

4. Surgery

In more severe cases, heart surgery may be required, such as valve repair or replacement, heart transplant, or the implantation of a pacemaker or defibrillator to regulate the heart's electrical activity.

5. Cardiac Rehabilitation

Following a heart event or procedure, cardiac rehabilitation programs can help individuals recover and adopt a heart-healthy lifestyle through exercise, education, and counseling.

Preventative measures and prompt detection are pivotal in diminishing the likelihood of heart disease and enhancing outcomes for individuals who have already received a diagnosis. Regular checkups with a healthcare provider and monitoring and addressing risk factors can significantly lower the chances of developing heart disease or experiencing complications.

Benefits of the Heart-Healthy Eating Pattern
A diet that is conducive to heart health can notably decrease the likelihood of developing heart disease or assist in regulating pre-existing conditions.

By focusing on nutrient-dense, minimally processed foods, a heart-healthy diet provides numerous benefits for overall health and well-being:

1. Lowering Blood Pressure And Cholesterol Levels

Blood pressure and LDL ("bad") cholesterol levels can be decreased with a heart-healthy diet that prioritizes nutrient-dense foods like fruits, vegetables, whole grains, lean proteins, and healthy fats. This diminishes the probability of plaque accumulation in the arteries.

2. Reducing Inflammation And Promoting Healthy Blood Flow

Antioxidants, which are found in foods like berries, leafy greens, and nuts, can help fight inflammation. Omega-3 fatty acids, which are found in fatty fish, flaxseeds, and walnuts, can help blood flow and keep the heart healthy.

3. Supporting a Healthy Weight

A heart-healthy eating pattern, combined with regular physical activity, can help maintain a healthy weight or promote weight loss, reducing the strain on the heart and decreasing the risk of heart disease.

4. Improving Blood Sugar Control

A well-balanced diet that is abundant in fiber and low in added sugars can aid in regulating blood sugar levels, which is especially crucial for individuals with diabetes or those susceptible to developing the disorder.

5. Strengthening The Immune System

A diet full of fruits, vegetables, and whole grains gives you vitamins, minerals, and antioxidants that boost your immune system and keep you from getting sick.

6. Reducing The Risk of Other Chronic Diseases

In addition to promoting heart health, a heart-healthy eating pattern can lower the risk of other chronic diseases, such as stroke, type 2 diabetes, and certain types of cancer.

7. Enhancing Mental Health And Cognitive Function

A heart-healthy diet can also benefit mental health and cognitive function by providing essential nutrients for brain health, such as omega-3 fatty acids, antioxidants, and B vitamins.

8. Promoting Healthy Digestion

A diet that is abundant in fiber sourced from fruits, vegetables, whole grains, and legumes can promote robust digestion, avert constipation, and diminish the likelihood of gastrointestinal ailments.

9. Boosting Energy Levels And Overall Well-Being

A well-balanced, heart-healthy eating pattern can provide sustained energy throughout the day and improve overall well-being by supplying the body with the essential nutrients it needs to function optimally.

Incorporating a heart-healthy dietary pattern not only diminishes the likelihood of heart disease but also yields a plethora of supplementary health advantages.

Tips and Tricks for Following a Healthy Eating Pattern

Adopting a heart-healthy eating pattern may seem challenging at first, but with a few simple tips and tricks, you can easily make sustainable changes to your diet and enjoy the benefits of a healthier lifestyle.

1. Plan Your Meals And Snacks

Create a weekly meal and snack schedule that incorporates a varied selection of nutrient-rich foods such as whole grains, lean proteins, fruits, vegetables, and healthy fats. This can help you make more intentional food choices and reduce the temptation to rely on unhealthy options.

For example, create a weekly meal plan and grocery list based on heart-healthy recipes that appeal to you. This will save you time and money and ensure you have the ingredients needed to prepare nutritious meals throughout the week.

2. Start with Small Changes

Instead of attempting to completely overhaul your eating habits all at once, gradually incorporate heart-healthy modifications into your diet. Small, manageable changes can make a big difference over time and are more likely to become lasting habits.

For example, add an extra serving of vegetables to your dinner, switch to whole-grain bread, or replace soda with water or herbal tea. This approach will help you build a heart-healthy eating pattern without feeling overwhelmed.

3. Practice Portion Control

Maintaining awareness of portion sizes can assist in preventing overconsumption and sustaining a healthy body weight. Use smaller plates and bowls to naturally reduce portion sizes, and pay attention to serving sizes listed on food labels. In addition, endeavor to consume food at a leisurely pace and pay attention to your body's indications of hunger and fullness.

You can do this by dividing your plate into sections, with half of the plate consisting of vegetables and fruits, one-quarter consisting of whole grains, and the remaining quarter containing lean proteins.

4. Cook at Home More Often

Preparing meals at home allows you to have better control over the ingredients and cooking methods used, ensuring that your meals are heart-healthy. Experiment with new recipes, and learn to modify your favorite dishes to make them healthier by reducing sodium, saturated fats, and added sugars. This will save you money and help you develop a deeper understanding of the nutritional content of your meals.

5. Make Healthier Swaps

Replace less healthy ingredients with more nutritious options in your everyday meals. For example, swap out white rice for brown rice or quinoa, use whole wheat pasta instead of regular pasta, and choose olive oil over butter or margarine. These simple swaps can significantly improve the nutritional quality of your meals without sacrificing taste.

6. Limit Processed Foods and Added Sugars

Restrict your consumption of processed foods, which are frequently high in sodium, unhealthy fats, and added sugars. Instead, focus on whole, minimally processed foods, and use natural sweeteners like honey or fruit to add sweetness to your meals and snacks.

7. Experiment with Herbs and Spices

Include a diverse array of herbs and spices in your culinary preparations to enhance taste without depending on salt or unhealthy fats. Experiment with various flavor combinations to discover your favorites, and keep a well-stocked spice cabinet to inspire heart-healthy culinary creativity.

8. Make Heart-Healthy Choices When Eating Out

When you're trying to eat heart-healthy, it can be hard to eat out, but with some planning and awareness, you can still enjoy restaurant meals without hurting your health. Choose dishes that are grilled, baked, or steamed, and ask for sauces and dressings to be served on the side. Avoid fried foods and dishes high in sodium, and choose whole-grain options when available.

9. Involve Family and Friends

Share your heart-healthy journey with your family and friends, and encourage them to join you in making healthier food choices. Cooking and eating together can provide support and accountability while making the experience more enjoyable and sustainable.

10. Be Patient and Persistent

Modifying your eating habits requires time, and it is essential to be patient with yourself as you establish a healthy dietary routine. Celebrate your successes, and remember that setbacks are a normal part of the process. Remain dedicated to your objectives and concentrate on the enduring advantages of a healthier way of life.

You can gradually establish a heart-healthy eating pattern that is both enjoyable and sustainable by using the following strategies. Embrace the process and keep in mind that even minor modifications can have a substantial impact on your overall health and well-being.

What to Eat and What to Avoid

When following a heart-healthy eating pattern, knowing which foods to include and which ones to limit or avoid is essential.

Here's a breakdown of what to eat and what to avoid, along with the health benefits and examples of each:

What to Eat:

1. Fruits and Vegetables

Fruits such as apples, berries, oranges, leafy greens, tomatoes, bell peppers, broccoli, and sweet potatoes are abundant in vitamins, minerals, antioxidants, and fiber, which can aid in lowering blood pressure, reducing inflammation, and promoting overall heart health. This category includes both fresh and frozen options, as well as dried fruits in moderation.

Strive to consume a minimum of 5 servings of fruits and vegetables each day, prioritizing a diverse range of colors and types. A standard serving size is usually equivalent to a moderate-sized fruit, 1/2 cup of cooked vegetables, or 1 cup of raw leafy greens.

2. Whole Grains

Whole grains are abundant in fiber, which can assist in lowering cholesterol levels and stabilizing blood sugar. Examples of whole grains comprise barley, brown rice, quinoa, whole wheat bread, and pasta. Furthermore, they contain essential nutrients such as B vitamins, iron, and magnesium, which promote heart health.

Strive for a minimum of three servings of whole grains per day. A single serving corresponds to 1/2 cup of cooked grains, one slice of whole wheat bread, or 1 cup of whole-grain cereal.

3. Lean Proteins

Choose lean protein sources like fish, tofu, beans, lentils, skinless poultry, and low-fat dairy items. Fish, particularly fatty varieties such as salmon, mackerel, and sardines, serve as an excellent source of omega-3 fatty acids that can mitigate inflammation and reinforce heart health. Due to their high fiber and plant-based protein content, beans and lentils can lower blood pressure and cholesterol levels.

Aim to consume 2-3 servings of lean protein per day, including at least two servings of fatty fish per week. One serving is equal to 3 ounces of cooked meat or poultry, 3/4 cup of cooked beans or lentils, or 1/4 cup of tofu.

4. Healthy Fats

Pick healthy fats like olive oil, nuts, seeds, and avocados. Monounsaturated and polyunsaturated fats, which are plentiful in these foods, can aid in reducing LDL cholesterol and decreasing inflammation. Nuts and seeds also provide essential nutrients like magnesium and vitamin E.

Strive for 2-3 servings of healthy fats per day. One serving is equivalent to 1/4 cup of nuts or seeds, 1/2 of a medium avocado, or 1 tablespoon of olive oil.

What to Avoid:

1. Saturated and Trans Fats

Incorporating saturated fats into one's diet in moderation is advised, as they are commonly found in full-fat dairy products, fatty meats, and tropical oils such as coconut and palm oil. In contrast, trans fats, which can elevate LDL cholesterol levels and heighten the risk of heart disease, can be found in partially hydrogenated oils and should be entirely avoided.

2. Excess Sodium

High blood pressure can be caused by too much sodium, so don't eat more than 2,300 milligrams (mg) of sodium every day. Limit processed foods, canned goods, and restaurant meals, often high in sodium, and opt for low-sodium or sodium-free products when available.

3. Added Sugars

Excessive consumption of added sugars can result in weight gain, inflammation, and elevated triglyceride levels, all of which are risk factors for heart disease. Limit consumption of sugary beverages, candies, baked goods, and other foods high in added sugars, and opt for naturally sweetened options like fruit.

4. Refined Carbohydrates

Reduce your intake of refined carbohydrates, which can lead to rapid blood sugar spikes and weight gain. Examples of these foods include white bread, white rice, and pastries. Instead, opt for whole-grain alternatives that are richer in nutrients and fiber.

By including nutrient-dense foods and limiting unhealthy options, you can create a healthy eating pattern that supports overall cardiovascular health and well-being. Additionally, keep in mind to monitor your portion sizes and relish a diverse range of foods to guarantee that you're fulfilling your nutritional requirements.

BREAKFAST RECIPES

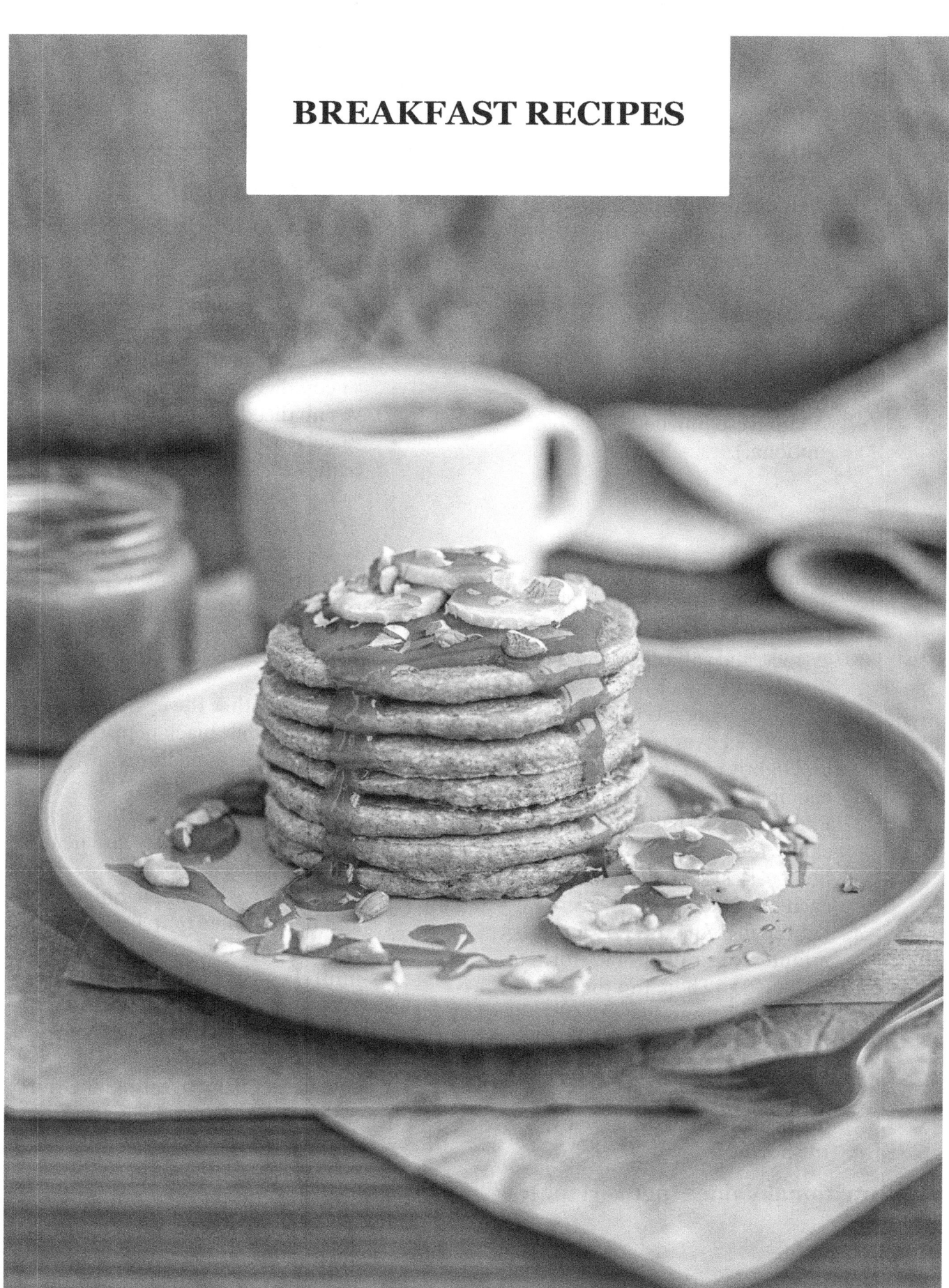

BANANA OAT PANCAKES

Ingredients:

- 1 ripe banana
- ½ cup old-fashioned oats
- ½ cup of unsweetened almond milk
- ¼ cup whole wheat flour
- ½ tsp baking powder
- ¼ tsp cinnamon
- ¼ tsp vanilla extract
- 1/8 tsp salt
- Non-stick cooking spray
- ¼ cup fresh blueberries (optional)

Instructions:

1. Combine banana, oats, almond milk, whole wheat flour, baking powder, cinnamon, vanilla extract, and salt in a blender. Blend until smooth.
2. Before cooking, preheat a non-stick skillet over medium heat and lightly coat it with non-stick cooking spray.
3. Pour ¼ cup of batter onto the skillet for each pancake. If using blueberries, sprinkle a few onto each pancake.
4. Let the ingredients cook for 2 to 3 minutes, or until bubbles form on the surface. Then, flip them over and cook for another 1 to 2 minutes, or until they turn golden brown.
5. Serve right away with your favorite toppings, like honey or fresh fruit.

Nutritional Values (per serving):

Calories: 245 | Fat: 3.5g | Saturated Fat: 0.5g | Cholesterol: 0mg | Sodium: 175mg | Carbohydrates: 47g | Fiber: 7g | Sugar: 9g | Protein: 8g

SPINACH AND MUSHROOM EGG WHITE SCRAMBLE

Ingredients:

- 4 large egg whites
- 1 cup baby spinach, chopped
- ½ cup mushrooms, sliced
- ¼ cup diced onion
- ¼ cup diced red bell pepper
- ¼ cup low-sodium feta cheese, crumbled
- ¼ tsp garlic powder
- ¼ tsp black pepper
- ¼ tsp dried basil
- Non-stick cooking spray

Instructions:

1. Whisk together the egg whites, garlic powder, black pepper, and dried basil in a medium bowl. Set aside.
2. Spray a nonstick pan with nonstick cooking spray and heat it to medium.
3. Take a pan and add the onions and bell peppers to it. Cook for approximately 3-4 minutes or until they start to become soft.
4. When the mushrooms are tender, add them back in and simmer for a further 3–4 minutes.
5. Add the spinach to the skillet and toss it in once the other ingredients have finished cooking. Cook the spinach for about 1-2 minutes, or until it has wilted.

6. After the vegetables are cooked, pour the egg white mixture over them in the skillet. Cook the mixture while occasionally stirring until the egg whites are fully cooked and no longer runny.
7. Remove from heat and sprinkle the low-sodium feta cheese over the top.
8. Serve immediately with whole-grain toast or a side of fresh fruit.

Nutritional Values (per serving):

Calories: 164 | Fat: 4g | Saturated Fat: 2g | Cholesterol: 10mg | Sodium: 290mg | Carbohydrates: 11g | Fiber: 3g | Sugar: 4g | Protein: 20g

OVERNIGHT CHIA PUDDING

Ingredients:

- ½ cup of unsweetened almond milk
- ½ cup plain Greek yogurt
- ¼ cup chia seeds
- ½ tsp vanilla extract
- ½ tsp honey
- ½ cup mixed berries (fresh or frozen)
- 2 tbsp chopped nuts (e.g., almonds, walnuts, or pecans)

Instructions:

1. Take a small bowl and whisk together the almond milk, Greek yogurt, chia seeds, vanilla extract, and honey until they are well combined.
2. Evenly distribute the mixture between two little jars or containers, then secure the lids.
3. Once you've mixed all the ingredients together, cover the bowl and put it in the fridge for at least 4 hours or overnight so the chia seeds can soak up the liquid and make the pudding thicker.
4. Top each pudding with mixed berries and chopped nuts when ready to serve.

Nutritional Values (per serving):

Calories: 250 | Fat: 13g | Saturated Fat: 1g | Cholesterol: 5mg | Sodium: 115mg | Carbohydrates: 24g | Fiber: 11g | Sugar: 8g | Protein: 12g

AVOCADO AND TOMATO TOAST

Ingredients:

- 2 slices whole-grain bread
- ½ ripe avocado
- ½ cup cherry tomatoes, halved
- ¼ tsp garlic powder
- ¼ tsp black pepper
- ¼ tsp red pepper flakes (optional)
- ¼ tsp dried basil
- ¼ tsp lemon juice

Instructions:

1. Toast the bread pieces until they are as crisp as you like.
2. Take a small bowl and mash the avocado in it using a fork. Add garlic powder, black pepper, and lemon juice to the mashed

avocado and mix until well combined.
3. On the toast slices, evenly distribute the mashed avocado.
4. Top each slice with halved cherry tomatoes and sprinkle with dried basil and red pepper flakes.
5. Serve immediately.

Nutritional Values (per serving):

Calories: 278 | Fat: 14g | Saturated Fat: 2g | Cholesterol: 0mg | Sodium: 260mg | Carbohydrates: 33g | Fiber: 9g | Sugar: 5g | Protein: 9g

APPLE CINNAMON QUINOA BREAKFAST BOWL

Ingredients:

- ¼ cup dry quinoa
- ½ cup water
- ¼ cup unsweetened almond milk
- ½ apple, diced
- ¼ tsp cinnamon
- ¼ tsp vanilla extract
- 1 tbsp chopped nuts (e.g., almonds, walnuts, or pecans)
- 1 tbsp dried cranberries

Instructions:

1. Start by heating up some water in a small saucepan until it boils.
2. When the water has boiled, add the quinoa and turn down the heat. When the quinoa has absorbed all the water and is fully cooked, add the water to the pot with the quinoa.
3. Cover the pot and let the mixture simmer for about 12 to 15 minutes.
4. Stir in the almond milk, diced apple, cinnamon, and vanilla extract, and cook for another 3-4 minutes until heated through.
5. Divide the quinoa mixture between two bowls and top with chopped nuts and dried cranberries.
6. Serve immediately.

Nutritional Values (per serving):

Calories: 235 | Fat: 7g | Saturated Fat: 1g | Cholesterol: 0mg | Sodium: 40mg | Carbohydrates: 38g | Fiber: 5g | Sugar: 9g | Protein: 6g

VEGGIE AND EGG BREAKFAST BURRITO

Ingredients:

- 2 whole wheat tortillas
- 4 large egg whites
- ¼ cup diced onion
- ¼ cup diced bell pepper
- ¼ cup diced tomato
- ¼ cup canned low-sodium black beans, rinsed and drained
- ¼ tsp ground cumin
- ¼ tsp black pepper
- ¼ cup shredded low-fat cheddar cheese
- Non-stick cooking spray

Instructions:

1. Whisk together the egg whites, ground cumin, and black pepper in a medium bowl. Set aside.

2. Lightly spritz a nonstick pan with nonstick cooking spray and heat it to medium.
3. Take a pan and add the onions and bell peppers to it. Cook for approximately 3-4 minutes or until they start to become soft.
4. When everything is hot, add the tomatoes and black beans, mix, and simmer for an additional 2–3 minutes.
5. After the vegetables are cooked, pour the egg white mixture over them in the skillet. Cook the mixture while occasionally stirring until the egg whites are fully cooked and no longer runny.
6. Heat the tortillas for 15-20 seconds in the microwave or for 1-2 minutes per side in a dry pan over low heat.
7. Divide the egg and vegetable mixture evenly between the two tortillas and sprinkle with shredded low-fat cheddar cheese.
8. To make a burrito, you roll up the dough and fold in the sides. Serve right away

Nutritional Values (per serving):

Calories: 285 | Fat: 6g | Saturated Fat: 2g | Cholesterol: 5mg | Sodium: 430mg | Carbohydrates: 38g | Fiber: 8g | Sugar: 4g | Protein: 20g

GREEK YOGURT AND BERRY PARFAIT

Ingredients:

- ½ cup mixed berries (fresh or frozen)
- ¼ cup low-fat granola
- 1 cup plain non-fat Greek yogurt
- ½ tsp honey

Instructions:

1. Put half of the Greek yogurt in a glass or bowl. Then add half of the mixed berries and half of the granola.
2. Repeat the layers with the remaining Greek yogurt, mixed berries, and granola.
3. Pour the honey on top, and serve it right away.

Nutritional Values (per serving):

Calories: 265 | Fat: 3g | Saturated Fat: 0g | Cholesterol: 5mg | Sodium: 80mg | Carbohydrates: 38g | Fiber: 5g | Sugar: 22g | Protein: 23g

PEANUT BUTTER AND BANANA SMOOTHIE

Ingredients:

- 1 ripe banana, sliced and frozen
- ½ cup of unsweetened almond milk
- ¼ cup plain non-fat Greek yogurt
- 1 tbsp natural peanut butter
- ½ tsp honey
- ¼ tsp vanilla extract
- ¼ cup ice (optional)

Instructions:

1. In a blender, combine the frozen banana slices, almond milk, Greek yogurt, peanut butter, honey, vanilla extract, and ice (if using). Mix until creamy and smooth.

2. Put the smoothie in two glasses right away and serve.

Nutritional Values (per serving):

Calories: 210 | Fat: 8g | Saturated Fat: 1g | Cholesterol: 0mg | Sodium: 135mg | Carbohydrates: 27g | Fiber: 3g | Sugar: 15g | Protein: 10g

VEGETABLE OMELET

Ingredients:

- 4 large egg whites
- ¼ cup diced bell pepper
- ¼ cup diced onion
- ¼ cup chopped mushrooms
- ¼ cup diced tomato
- ¼ cup chopped baby spinach
- ¼ tsp garlic powder
- ¼ tsp black pepper
- ¼ cup shredded low-fat cheddar cheese
- Non-stick cooking spray

Instructions:

1. Begin by taking a medium-sized bowl and whisking together the garlic powder, black pepper, and egg whites. Set the mixture aside so you can use it later. Next, heat a pan that doesn't stick on medium heat. Spray the skillet with nonstick cooking spray sparingly. The onions and bell peppers should now be added to the skillet and cooked for 3–4 minutes, or until they begin to soften. The mushrooms should be added to the skillet and cooked for an additional 3–4 minutes, or until they are tender.
2. Cook the tomatoes and baby spinach, stirring occasionally, for 1-2 minutes, or until the spinach wilts.
3. When the vegetables are done, pour the egg white mixture over them in the skillet. The mixture is ready when the edges begin to set but the center is still a little runny, which takes about 3 to 4 minutes.
4. One half of the omelet should be covered with low-fat cheddar cheese crumbles. The other half should be folded over the cheese carefully.
5. Cook the omelet for a further 1-2 minutes, or until the cheese is melted and the omelet is done.
6. Split the omelet in half, then serve right away.

Nutritional Values (per serving):

Calories: 140 | Fat: 2g | Saturated Fat: 1g | Cholesterol: 5mg | Sodium: 280mg | Carbohydrates: 11g | Fiber: 3g | Sugar: 4g | Protein: 18g

BERRY OATMEAL

Ingredients:

- 1 cup old-fashioned oats
- 2 cups water
- ¼ tsp cinnamon
- ¼ tsp vanilla extract
- ½ cup mixed berries (fresh or frozen)
- 1 tbsp chopped nuts (e.g., almonds, walnuts, or pecans)
- ½ tsp honey

Instructions:

1. Bring the water to a boil in a medium-sized pot. Put the oats in the pot, and turn the heat down to low. Simmer the oats for 5-7 minutes, occasionally stirring, until they become tender and have absorbed all the water.
2. Stir in the cinnamon and vanilla extract.
3. Separate the oats evenly into two bowls and add a mixture of berries, chopped nuts, and a slight drizzle of honey on top of each.
4. Serve immediately.

Nutritional Values (per serving):

Calories: 230 | Fat: 6g | Saturated Fat: 1g | Cholesterol: 0mg | Sodium: 10mg | Carbohydrates: 38g | Fiber: 6g | Sugar: 8g | Protein: 7g

TROPICAL GREEN SMOOTHIE

Ingredients:

- 1 cup baby spinach
- ½ cup frozen pineapple chunks
- ½ cup frozen mango chunks
- ½ banana, sliced and frozen
- 1 cup unsweetened almond milk
- ¼ cup plain non-fat Greek yogurt
- ½ tsp honey

Instructions:

1. In a blender, combine the baby spinach, frozen pineapple chunks, frozen mango chunks, frozen banana slices, almond milk, Greek yogurt, and honey. Blend until smooth and creamy.
2. Once the smoothie is blended to your desired consistency, divide it evenly into two glasses and serve immediately.

Nutritional Values (per serving):

Calories: 150 | Fat: 2g | Saturated Fat: 0g | Cholesterol: 0mg | Sodium: 120mg | Carbohydrates: 30g | Fiber: 4g | Sugar: 21g | Protein: 7g

COTTAGE CHEESE AND FRUIT BOWL

Ingredients:

- 1 cup low-fat cottage cheese
- ½ cup mixed fruit (e.g., berries, diced peaches, or pineapple)
- ¼ cup low-fat granola
- 1 tbsp chopped nuts (e.g., almonds, walnuts, or pecans)
- ½ tsp honey

Instructions:

1. Put the oats in the pot, and turn the heat down to low.
2. Top each bowl with mixed fruit, low-fat granola, chopped nuts, and a drizzle of honey.
3. Serve immediately.

Nutritional Values (per serving):

Calories: 255 | Fat: 6g | Saturated Fat: 1g | Cholesterol: 10mg | Sodium: 380mg | Carbohydrates: 32g | Fiber: 3g | Sugar: 20g | Protein: 20g

MULTIGRAIN WAFFLES WITH FRUIT

Ingredients:

- 2 frozen multigrain waffles
- ½ cup mixed berries (fresh or frozen)
- ¼ cup plain non-fat Greek yogurt
- ½ tsp honey
- ¼ tsp ground cinnamon

Instructions:

1. Toast the frozen multigrain waffles according to the package directions.
2. Mix the Greek yogurt, honey, and cinnamon in a small bowl.
3. Top each waffle with half of the yogurt mixture and a portion of mixed berries.
4. Serve immediately.

Nutritional Values (per serving):

Calories: 240 | Fat: 7g | Saturated Fat: 1g | Cholesterol: 0mg | Sodium: 380mg | Carbohydrates: 36g | Fiber: 5g | Sugar: 11g | Protein: 10g

ALMOND BUTTER AND APPLE RICE CAKES

Ingredients:

- 2 brown rice cakes
- 2 tbsp natural almond butter
- ½ apple, thinly sliced
- ¼ tsp ground cinnamon

Instructions:

1. Spread 1 tbsp of almond butter onto each rice cake.
2. Place the apple slices on top of the almond butter, making sure there are equal amounts on each rice cake.
3. Dust the apple slices with cinnamon powder.

Nutritional Values (per serving):

Calories: 235 | Fat: 12g | Saturated Fat: 1g | Cholesterol: 0mg | Sodium: 45mg | Carbohydrates: 28g | Fiber: 4g | Sugar: 9g | Protein: 6g

SPINACH, TOMATO, AND MOZZARELLA FRITTATA

Ingredients:

- 4 large egg whites
- ½ cup of baby spinach, chopped
- ½ cup cherry tomatoes, halved
- ¼ cup shredded low-fat mozzarella cheese
- ¼ tsp garlic powder
- ¼ tsp black pepper
- ¼ tsp dried basil
- Non-stick cooking spray

Instructions:

1. Whisk the egg whites, garlic powder, black pepper, and dried basil together in a medium-sized bowl until everything is well-mixed. Don't use the bowl.
2. Before starting to cook, preheat the oven to 375°F (190°C).
3. Place an oven-safe nonstick skillet over medium heat and

lightly spray it with nonstick cooking spray.
4. Include the baby spinach in the pan and cook for roughly one to two minutes or until it becomes tender.
5. Cook for another 1-2 minutes after adding the cherry tomatoes.
6. Pour the egg white mixture over the spinach in the skillet and cook for approximately 3 to 4 minutes, until the edges are set but the center is still runny.
7. Shred low-fat mozzarella cheese and sprinkled it on top of the frittata.
8. Put the pan in a hot oven for 8 to 10 minutes, or until the cheese is melted and the frittata is done.
9. Take the frittata out of the oven, wait a minute for it to cool, and then cut it in half. Serve right away.

Nutritional Values (per serving):

Calories: 125 | Fat: 2g | Saturated Fat: 1g | Cholesterol: 5mg | Sodium: 270mg | Carbohydrates: 6g | Fiber: 1g | Sugar: 3g | Protein:18g

SMOKED SALMON AND AVOCADO RICE CAKE

Ingredients:

- 2 brown rice cakes
- ¼ cup mashed avocado
- ¼ tsp black pepper
- ¼ tsp lemon juice
- 2 oz smoked salmon
- ¼ cup cucumber, thinly sliced
- 1 tbsp capers (optional)

Instructions:

1. In a small bowl, mix together the mashed avocado, black pepper, and lemon juice.
2. On the rice cakes, evenly distribute the avocado mixture.
3. Each rice cake should have smoked salmon and cucumber slices on top.
4. Optionally, sprinkle capers over the top.
5. Serve immediately.

Nutritional Values (per serving):

Calories: 250 | Fat: 12g | Saturated Fat: 2g | Cholesterol: 10mg | Sodium: 720mg | Carbohydrates: 23g | Fiber: 3g | Sugar: 1g | Protein: 14g

TURKEY SAUSAGE AND VEGGIE SCRAMBLE

Ingredients:

- 2 turkey sausage links, cooked and sliced
- ½ cup chopped bell pepper
- ½ cup chopped onion
- ½ cup chopped mushrooms
- ½ cup chopped zucchini
- 4 large egg whites
- ¼ tsp garlic powder
- ¼ tsp black pepper
- Non-stick cooking spray

Instructions:

1. Whisk together the egg whites, garlic powder, and black pepper in a medium bowl. Set aside.

2. Coat a nonstick skillet lightly with cooking spray and heat it over medium heat.
3. Take a pan and add the onions and peppers to it. Cook for approximately 3-4 minutes or until they start to become soft.
4. Add the mushrooms and zucchini and cook for another 3–4 minutes, until the vegetables are soft.
5. Incorporate the cooked turkey sausage slices into the mixture and cook for 1-2 minutes until thoroughly heated.
6. After the vegetables and sausage are cooked, pour the egg-white mixture over them in the skillet. Cook for approximately 3-4 minutes while lifting the edges occasionally to allow the uncooked egg to flow underneath. Keep cooking the omelet until it is done all the way through and no longer wet.
7. The scramble should be split between two plates and served right away.

Nutritional Values (per serving):

Calories: 200 | Fat: 6g | Saturated Fat: 1g | Cholesterol: 35mg | Sodium: 450mg | Carbohydrates: 15g | Fiber: 3g | Sugar: 5g | Protein: 22g

CHIA PUDDING WITH FRUIT

Ingredients:

- ¼ cup chia seeds
- 1 cup unsweetened almond milk
- ½ tsp vanilla extract
- ½ tsp honey
- ½ cup mixed fruit (e.g., berries, diced peaches, or pineapple)

Instructions:

1. Combine the chia seeds, almond milk, vanilla extract, and honey in a small bowl or jar.
2. Cover the bowl or jar and place it in the refrigerator overnight, or for a minimum of 4 hours, until the chia seeds have absorbed the liquid and the mixture has attained the consistency of pudding.
3. When the pudding is ready to be served, divide it between two bowls or jars. Top each with a portion of mixed fruit and serve immediately.

Nutritional Values (per serving):

Calories: 180 | Fat: 8g | Saturated Fat: 1g | Cholesterol: 0mg | Sodium: 100mg | Carbohydrates: 21g | Fiber: 10g | Sugar: 9g | Protein: 6g

GREEK YOGURT WITH GRANOLA AND BERRIES

Ingredients:

- 1 cup non-fat plain Greek yogurt
- ¼ cup low-fat granola
- ½ cup mixed berries (e.g., blueberries, raspberries, or strawberries)
- 1 tsp honey (optional)

Instructions:

1. Divide the Greek yogurt between two bowls.
2. Top each bowl with half of the granola and mixed berries.
3. Optionally, drizzle each bowl with honey before serving.

Nutritional Values (per serving):

Calories: 195 | Fat: 2g | Saturated Fat: 0g | Cholesterol: 5mg | Sodium: 60mg | Carbohydrates: 30g | Fiber: 3g | Sugar: 18g | Protein: 16g

AVOCADO AND EGG TOAST

Ingredients:

- 2 slices whole-grain bread
- ½ avocado, mashed
- ¼ tsp black pepper
- ¼ tsp lemon juice
- 2 large eggs
- Non-stick cooking spray

Instructions:

1. Toast the whole-grain bread slices.
2. Mix the mashed avocado, black pepper, and lemon juice in a small bowl.
3. Heat a nonstick skillet over medium-high heat. Apply a thin layer of nonstick cooking spray to the skillet. Gently break the eggs and add them to the pan, cooking until they reach your preferred level of doneness.
4. Spread the avocado mixture onto the toast slices, then top each with a cooked egg.
5. Serve immediately.

Nutritional Values (per serving):

Calories: 320 | Fat: 18g | Saturated Fat: 3g | Cholesterol: 185mg | Sodium: 310mg | Carbohydrates: 27g | Fiber: 7g | Sugar: 4g | Protein: 15g

PINEAPPLE, BANANA, AND SPINACH SMOOTHIE

Ingredients:

- 1 cup fresh or frozen pineapple chunks
- 1 ripe banana
- 1 cup baby spinach
- ½ cup unsweetened almond milk
- ½ cup non-fat plain Greek yogurt
- 1 tbsp honey (optional)

Instructions:

1. Blend the pineapple, banana, spinach, almond milk, Greek yogurt, and honey (if desired) together until the mixture is smooth.
2. Immediately after blending, transfer the contents of the smoothie into two glasses and serve promptly.

Nutritional Values (per serving):

Calories: 190 | Fat: 1g | Saturated Fat: 0g | Cholesterol: 0mg | Sodium: 110mg | Carbohydrates: 40g | Fiber: 4g | Sugar: 27g | Protein: 8g

QUINOA AND BERRY BREAKFAST BOWL

Ingredients:

- ½ cup cooked quinoa
- ½ cup mixed berries (e.g., blueberries, raspberries, or strawberries)
- ¼ cup non-fat plain Greek yogurt
- 1 tbsp chopped nuts (e.g., almonds, walnuts, or pecans)
- 1 tsp honey (optional)

Instructions:

1. Divide the cooked quinoa between two bowls.
2. Greek yogurt, chopped nuts, and half of the mixed berries should be placed on top of each bowl.
3. Optionally, drizzle each bowl with honey before serving.

Nutritional Values (per serving):

Calories: 210 | Fat: 4g | Saturated Fat: 0g | Cholesterol: 0mg | Sodium: 30mg | Carbohydrates: 34g | Fiber: 5g | Sugar: 11g | Protein: 11g

GREEN DETOX SMOOTHIE

Ingredients:

- 1 cup baby spinach
- ½ cucumber chopped
- ½ green apple chopped
- ½ cup fresh or frozen pineapple chunks
- ½ cup unsweetened almond milk
- ½ cup water
- ½ cup ice (optional)

Instructions:

1. In a blender, combine the spinach, cucumber, green apple, pineapple, almond milk, water, and ice (if using). Blend until smooth.
2. Blend the ingredients until smooth, then pour the smoothie into two glasses and serve immediately.

Nutritional Values (per serving):

Calories: 80 | Fat: 1g | Saturated Fat: 0g | Cholesterol: 0mg | Sodium: 70mg | Carbohydrates: 17g | Fiber: 3g | Sugar: 11g | Protein: 2g

VEGGIE AND HUMMUS WRAP

Ingredients:

- 2 whole-grain tortillas
- ¼ cup hummus
- ½ cup shredded lettuce
- ½ cup chopped bell pepper
- ½ cup chopped cucumber
- ½ cup grated carrot

Instructions:

1. Lay the whole-grain tortillas on a flat surface.
2. Spread half of the hummus on each tortilla.
3. Top each tortilla with half of the shredded lettuce, bell pepper, cucumber, and grated carrot.
4. Roll the tortillas firmly, folding in the sides as you proceed.
5. Each wrap should be cut in half and served right away.

Nutritional Values (per serving):

Calories: 220 | Fat: 7g | Saturated Fat: 1g | Cholesterol: 0mg | Sodium: 400mg | Carbohydrates: 34g | Fiber: 7g | Sugar: 5g | Protein: 8g

---

COTTAGE CHEESE AND FRUIT BOWL

Ingredients:

- 1 cup low-fat cottage cheese
- ½ cup mixed fruit (e.g., berries, diced peaches, or pineapple)
- 1 tbsp chopped nuts (e.g., almonds, walnuts, or pecans)
- 1 tsp honey (optional)

Instructions:

1. The cottage cheese should be split between two bowls.
2. Top each bowl with half of the mixed fruit and chopped nuts.
3. Optionally, drizzle each bowl with honey before serving.

Nutritional Values (per serving):

Calories: 180 | Fat: 4g | Saturated Fat: 1g | Cholesterol: 5mg | Sodium: 400mg | Carbohydrates: 20g | Fiber: 2g | Sugar: 15g | Protein: 16g

SNACK RECIPES

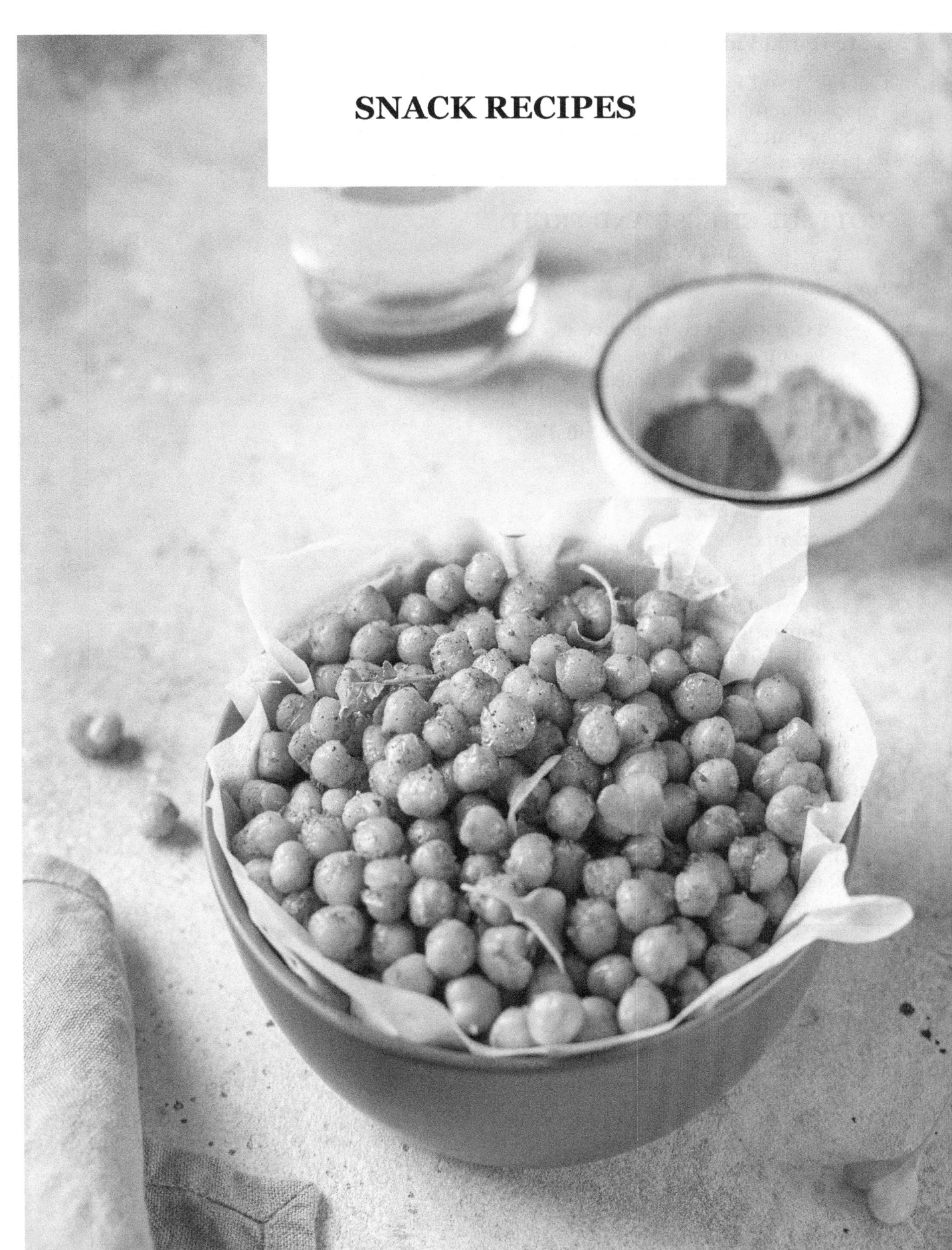

SPICY ROASTED CHICKPEAS

Ingredients:

- 1 (15 oz) can of chickpeas, drained, rinsed, and patted dry
- 1 tbsp olive oil
- ¼ tsp paprika
- ¼ tsp garlic powder
- ¼ tsp cayenne pepper
- ¼ tsp salt

Instructions:

1. Set the oven's temperature to 400°F (200°C). Cover a baking sheet with parchment paper.
2. In a bowl, mix the chickpeas, olive oil, paprika, garlic powder, cayenne pepper, and salt.
3. Spread the chickpeas in a single layer on the baking sheet that has been ready.
4. Bake until crispy and golden brown, shaking the pan once halfway through, for approximately 30-35 minutes.
5. Let the chickpeas cool down a bit before you serve them. Keep leftovers in a container that doesn't let air in.

Nutritional Values (per serving):

Calories: 130 | Fat: 5g | Saturated Fat: 0.5g | Cholesterol: 0mg | Sodium: 250mg | Carbohydrates: 17g | Fiber: 5g | Sugar: 3g | Protein: 6g

GREEK YOGURT RANCH DIP WITH VEGGIES

Ingredients:

- 1 cup non-fat plain Greek yogurt
- 1 tbsp dry ranch dressing mix
- 2 cups mixed vegetables (e.g., baby carrots, celery sticks, cucumber slices, or cherry tomatoes)

Instructions:

1. Mix the Greek yogurt and dry ranch dressing mix together in a small bowl.
2. Divide the Greek yogurt ranch dip and mixed vegetables between two plates.
3. Serve immediately.

Nutritional Values (per serving):

Calories: 110 | Fat: 0g | Saturated Fat: 0g | Cholesterol: 5mg | Sodium: 430mg | Carbohydrates: 14g | Fiber: 3g | Sugar: 7g | Protein: 12g

APPLE SLICES WITH ALMOND BUTTER

Ingredients:

- 1 large apple, cored and sliced
- 2 tbsp almond butter

Instructions:

1. Divide the apple slices between two plates.
2. Serve each plate with 1 tablespoon of almond butter for dipping.

Nutritional Values (per serving):

Calories: 190 | Fat: 10g | Saturated Fat: 1g | Cholesterol: 0mg | Sodium: 0mg |

Carbohydrates: 24g | Fiber: 5g | Sugar: 17g | Protein: 4g

MINI CAPRESE SKEWERS

Ingredients:

- 10 cherry tomatoes
- 10 small fresh mozzarella balls
- 10 fresh basil leaves
- 1 tbsp balsamic glaze

Instructions:

1. Thread a cherry tomato, mozzarella ball, and basil leaf onto each of the 10 small skewers.
2. Before serving, put the skewers on a plate and drizzle them with balsamic glaze.

Nutritional Values (per serving):

Calories: 150 | Fat: 9g | Saturated Fat: 5g | Cholesterol: 30mg | Sodium: 200mg | Carbohydrates: 9g | Fiber: 1g | Sugar: 7g | Protein: 9g

CELERY STICKS WITH CREAM CHEESE AND EVERYTHING BAGEL SEASONING

Ingredients:

- 4 celery stalks cut into 3-inch sticks
- ¼ cup low-fat cream cheese
- 1 tbsp everything bagel seasoning

Instructions:

1. Fill the celery sticks with cream cheese.
2. Everything bagel seasoning should be put on the celery sticks that have been filled.
3. The celery sticks should be divided between two plates and served.

Nutritional Values (per serving):

Calories: 80 | Fat: 4g | Saturated Fat: 2.5g | Cholesterol: 15mg | Sodium: 320mg | Carbohydrates: 6g | Fiber: 1g | Sugar: 2g | Protein: 4g

AVOCADO-STUFFED CHERRY TOMATOES

Ingredients:

- 12 cherry tomatoes
- 1 ripe avocado, mashed
- ¼ tsp garlic powder
- ¼ tsp black pepper
- ¼ tsp lemon juice

Instructions:

1. Slice the tops of the cherry tomatoes and carefully scoop out the insides with a small spoon.
2. Mix the mashed avocado, garlic powder, black pepper, and lemon juice in a small bowl.
3. Use a small spoon or a piping bag to put the avocado mixture into the cherry tomatoes.
4. The stuffed cherry tomatoes should be divided between two plates and served.

Nutritional Values (per serving):

Calories: 130 | Fat: 10g | Saturated Fat: 1.5g | Cholesterol: 0mg | Sodium: 25mg

| Carbohydrates: 10g | Fiber: 4g | Sugar: 4g | Protein: 2g

CUCUMBER SLICES WITH HUMMUS

Ingredients:

- 1 large cucumber, sliced
- ¼ cup hummus

Instructions:

1. Divide the cucumber slices between two plates.
2. Serve each plate with 2 tablespoons of hummus for dipping.

Nutritional Values (per serving):

Calories: 80 | Fat: 4g | Saturated Fat: 0.5g | Cholesterol: 0mg | Sodium: 180mg | Carbohydrates: 10g | Fiber: 2g | Sugar: 2g | Protein: 4g

ANTS ON A LOG

Ingredients:

- 4 celery stalks cut into 3-inch sticks
- 2 tbsp peanut butter
- 2 tbsp raisins

Instructions:

1. Fill the celery sticks with peanut butter.
2. Press the raisins into the peanut butter on each celery stick.
3. Divide the ants on a log between two plates and serve.

Nutritional Values (per serving):

Calories: 170 | Fat: 9g | Saturated Fat: 2g | Cholesterol: 0mg | Sodium: 115mg | Carbohydrates: 20g | Fiber: 2g | Sugar: 12g | Protein: 5g

EASY EDAMAME

Ingredients:

- 1 cup frozen shelled edamame
- ¼ tsp salt
- ¼ tsp black pepper

Instructions:

1. Cook the edamame according to the package instructions, usually by boiling or steaming for 3-5 minutes.
2. After draining the edamame, sprinkle with salt and black pepper to taste.
3. Divide the edamame between two plates and serve warm.

Nutritional Values (per serving):

Calories: 100 | Fat: 4g | Saturated Fat: 0.5g | Cholesterol: 0mg | Sodium: 310mg | Carbohydrates: 9g | Fiber: 4g | Sugar: 2g | Protein: 8g

PEANUT BUTTER AND CHOCOLATE RICE CAKES

Ingredients:

- 2 brown rice cakes
- 2 tbsp peanut butter
- 2 tsp chocolate chips

Instructions:

1. On each rice cake, spread 1 tablespoon of peanut butter.
2. Sprinkle each rice cake with 1 teaspoon of chocolate chips.
3. Serve immediately.

Nutritional Values (per serving):

Calories: 210 | Fat: 11g | Saturated Fat: 2.5g | Cholesterol: 0mg | Sodium: 75mg | Carbohydrates: 23g | Fiber: 1g | Sugar: 8g | Protein: 5g

SPINACH AND ARTICHOKE DIP

Ingredients:

- ½ cup non-fat plain Greek yogurt
- ½ cup canned artichoke hearts, drained and chopped
- ½ cup chopped spinach (fresh or thawed frozen)
- ¼ cup grated Parmesan cheese
- ¼ tsp garlic powder
- ¼ tsp black pepper
- Whole grain crackers or raw veggies for serving

Instructions:

1. Combine Greek yogurt, artichoke hearts, spinach, Parmesan cheese, garlic powder, and black pepper in a medium-sized bowl.
2. Serve the dip with whole grain crackers or raw veggies.

Nutritional Values (per serving):

Calories: 100 | Fat: 3g | Saturated Fat: 1.5g | Cholesterol: 10mg | Sodium: 320mg | Carbohydrates: 7g | Fiber: 1g | Sugar: 3g | Protein: 11g

FRUIT KABOBS WITH HONEY-YOGURT DRIP

Ingredients:

- 1 cup mixed fruit (e.g., berries, grapes, pineapple, or kiwi)
- ½ cup non-fat plain Greek yogurt
- 1 tbsp honey

Instructions:

1. Thread the mixed fruit onto 4 skewers.
2. Mix the Greek yogurt and honey in a small bowl.
3. Divide the fruit kabobs and honey-yogurt dip between two plates and serve.

Nutritional Values (per serving):

Calories: 120 | Fat: 0g | Saturated Fat: 0g | Cholesterol: 0mg | Sodium: 25mg | Carbohydrates: 26g | Fiber: 2g | Sugar: 22g | Protein: 6g

SLICED TURKEY AND CHEESE ROLL-UPS

Ingredients:

- 4 slices low-sodium deli turkey
- 2 slices reduced-fat Swiss cheese, halved
- 4 large lettuce leaves

Instructions:

1. Lay a lettuce leaf on a flat surface.
2. Place a slice of deli turkey on the lettuce leaf.
3. Top the turkey with a half slice of Swiss cheese.
4. Tightly roll the lettuce leaf, tucking the sides in as you go.
5. Repeat steps 1-4 with the remaining ingredients.
6. Divide the turkey and cheese roll-ups between two plates and serve.

Nutritional Values (per serving):

Calories: 100 | Fat: 4g | Saturated Fat: 2g | Cholesterol: 30mg | Sodium: 380mg | Carbohydrates: 2g | Fiber: 0g | Sugar: 1g | Protein: 14g

POPCORN WITH NUTRITIONAL YEAST

Ingredients:

- 3 cups air-popped popcorn
- 1 tbsp olive oil
- 2 tbsp nutritional yeast
- ¼ tsp salt

Instructions:

1. Drizzle the olive oil over the popcorn and toss to coat.
2. Sprinkle the nutritional yeast and salt over the popcorn, and toss again to distribute the seasonings evenly.
3. Divide the popcorn between two bowls and serve.

Nutritional Values (per serving):

Calories: 120 | Fat: 7g | Saturated Fat: 1g | Cholesterol: 0mg | Sodium: 300mg | Carbohydrates: 10g | Fiber: 2g | Sugar: 0g | Protein: 4g

BELL PEPPER NACHOS

Ingredients:

- 1 large bell pepper, sliced into thin strips
- ¼ cup black beans rinsed and drained
- ¼ cup shredded reduced-fat cheddar cheese
- 2 tbsp diced tomatoes
- 2 tbsp diced avocado

Instructions:

1. Set the oven's temperature to 400°F (200°C). Cover a baking sheet with parchment paper.
2. Put one layer of bell pepper slices on the baking sheet.
3. Top the bell pepper slices with black beans and shredded cheddar cheese.
4. For 5–7 minutes, bake the cheese until it melts and starts to bubble.
5. When it comes out of the oven, put diced avocado and tomato on top.
6. The nachos with bell peppers should be split between two plates and served.

Nutritional Values (per serving):

Calories: 130 | Fat: 6g | Saturated Fat: 2g | Cholesterol: 10mg | Sodium: 180mg | Carbohydrates: 13g | Fiber: 4g | Sugar: 3g | Protein: 8g

VEGGIE PINWHEELS

Ingredients:

- 1 large whole wheat tortilla
- 2 tbsp reduced-fat cream cheese
- ½ cup mixed vegetables (e.g., shredded carrots, cucumber, or bell pepper)

Instructions:

1. Spread the cream cheese on the whole wheat tortilla.
2. Arrange the mixed vegetables on the tortilla.
3. Roll the tortilla tightly and slice it into 1-inch pinwheels.
4. Place two pinwheels on each of two plates and serve.

Nutritional Values (per serving):

Calories: 110 | Fat: 3g | Saturated Fat: 1g | Cholesterol: 10mg | Sodium: 260mg | Carbohydrates: 16g | Fiber: 2g | Sugar: 2g | Protein: 4g

FROZEN YOGURT BARK

Ingredients:

- 1 cup non-fat plain Greek yogurt
- 1 tbsp honey
- ¼ cup mixed berries
- 1 tbsp chopped nuts (e.g., almonds, walnuts, or pecans)

Instructions:

1. Line a baking sheet with parchment paper.
2. Mix the Greek yogurt and honey in a small bowl.
3. Evenly spread the yogurt mixture onto the prepared baking sheet in a thin layer.
4. Scatter the mixed berries and chopped nuts over the yogurt layer.
5. Place in the freezer for a minimum of 2 hours or until the mixture becomes firm.
6. Split the frozen yogurt bark into pieces and put them on two plates in an even way. Serve immediately.

Nutritional Values (per serving):

Calories: 150 | Fat: 4g | Saturated Fat: 0.5g | Cholesterol: 0mg | Sodium: 45mg | Carbohydrates: 18g | Fiber: 1g | Sugar: 15g | Protein: 12g

CHOCOLATE BANANA BITES

Ingredients:

- 1 large banana, sliced
- 2 tbsp dark chocolate chips
- 1 tsp coconut oil

Instructions:

1. Line a plate or baking sheet with parchment paper.
2. Mix the dark chocolate chips and coconut oil in a small bowl that can go in the microwave. Heat the chocolate in the microwave in 15-second intervals, pausing to stir between each interval, until it has melted and become smooth. Dip each banana slice into the melted chocolate, letting the excess drip

off, and place it on the prepared plate.
3. Freeze the chocolate-covered banana slices for at least 1 hour or until firm.
4. Serve the frozen banana bites by dividing them between two plates.

Nutritional Values (per serving):

Calories: 150 | Fat: 7g | Saturated Fat: 5g | Cholesterol: 0mg | Sodium: 0mg | Carbohydrates: 23g | Fiber: 2g | Sugar: 15g | Protein: 1g

SMOKED SALMON AND CREAM CHEESE CUCUMBER BITES

Ingredients:

- 1 large cucumber, sliced
- 4 oz smoked salmon, cut into small pieces
- ¼ cup reduced-fat cream cheese
- 1 tbsp chopped fresh dill

Instructions:

1. Top each cucumber slice with a small piece of smoked salmon.
2. Dollop a small amount of cream cheese onto each smoked salmon-topped cucumber slice.
3. Sprinkle a little fresh dill on each bite of cucumber.
4. Serve the cucumber bites by dividing them between two plates.

Nutritional Values (per serving):

Calories: 100 | Fat: 4g | Saturated Fat: 2g | Cholesterol: 20mg | Sodium: 430mg | Carbohydrates: 4g | Fiber: 1g | Sugar: 2g | Protein: 11g

CHEESE AND CRACKERS

Ingredients:

- 2 oz reduced-fat cheddar cheese, sliced
- 10 whole grain crackers

Instructions:

1. Divide the cheese slices and whole-grain crackers between two plates.
2. Serve immediately.

Nutritional Values (per serving):

Calories: 150 | Fat: 6g | Saturated Fat: 3g | Cholesterol: 15mg | Sodium: 250mg | Carbohydrates: 14g | Fiber: 2g | Sugar: 2g | Protein: 9g

MEAT RECIPES

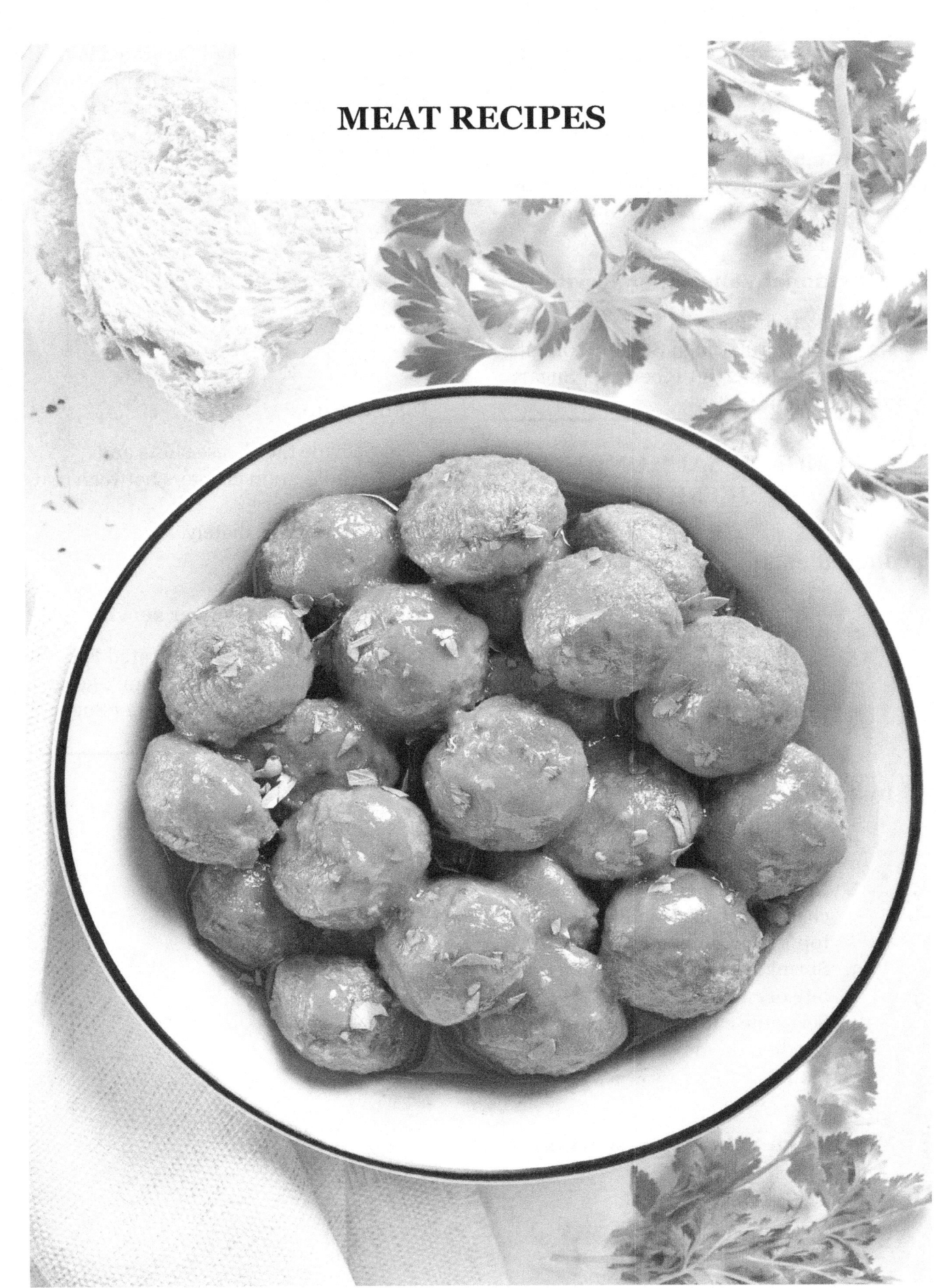

TURKEY MEATBALLS

Ingredients:

- ½ lb lean ground turkey
- ¼ cup whole wheat breadcrumbs
- ¼ cup grated Parmesan cheese
- ¼ cup chopped fresh parsley
- ¼ tsp garlic powder
- ¼ tsp salt
- ¼ tsp black pepper
- 1 large egg, beaten
- 1 tbsp olive oil

Instructions:

1. Mix the ground turkey, breadcrumbs, chopped mushrooms, diced onion, salt, black pepper, and beaten egg together in a large bowl. Mix until everything is well blended.
2. Make 8 even-sized meatballs from the mixture.
3. Heat the olive oil on medium heat in a non-stick pan. Add the meatballs to the pan and cook for 8-10 minutes, flipping occasionally, until they are browned on all sides and fully cooked.
4. Serve the turkey meatballs with your favorite marinara sauce or on top of whole wheat spaghetti.

Nutritional Values (per serving):

Calories: 250 | Fat: 13g | Saturated Fat: 4g | Cholesterol: 105mg | Sodium: 460mg | Carbohydrates: 8g | Fiber: 1g | Sugar: 1g | Protein: 24g

PORK TENDERLOIN WITH BALSAMIC GLAZE

Ingredients:

- ½ lb pork tenderloin, trimmed of excess fat
- ¼ tsp salt
- ¼ tsp black pepper
- 1 tbsp olive oil
- ¼ cup balsamic vinegar
- ¼ cup low-sodium chicken broth
- 1 tbsp honey

Instructions:

1. Set the oven to 375°F (190°C) and turn it on.
2. Season the pork tenderloin with salt and black pepper to taste.
3. Heat the olive oil in an oven-safe pan on medium-high heat. Place the pork tenderloin in the pan and cook each side for 2-3 minutes or until browned.
4. Roast the pork in the skillet in the oven for about 20 minutes, or until it is done.
5. While the pork is cooking, prepare the balsamic glaze by combining the balsamic vinegar, chicken broth, and honey in a small saucepan. Allow the sauce to simmer on medium heat until it has reduced by half and thickened.
6. Let the pork cool completely before slicing it.
7. Drizzle the balsamic glaze over the sliced pork and serve.

Nutritional Values (per serving):

Calories: 280 | Fat: 12g | Saturated Fat: 2.5g | Cholesterol: 80mg | Sodium:

420mg | Carbohydrates: 12g | Fiber: 0g | Sugar: 10g | Protein: 29g

BEEF STIR-FRY WITH BROCCOLI

Ingredients:

- ½ lb lean beef sirloin, thinly sliced
- ¼ tsp salt
- ¼ tsp black pepper
- 1 tbsp olive oil
- 1 cup broccoli florets
- ¼ cup low-sodium soy sauce
- ¼ cup water
- ½ tbsp cornstarch
- ½ tbsp honey
- ½ tsp minced garlic
- ½ tsp grated fresh ginger

Instructions:

1. Season the beef slices with salt and black pepper.
2. Heat a large nonstick skillet over medium-high heat with olive oil. Add the beef to the skillet and cook for 2-3 minutes on each side until it is browned. Get the beef out of the pan and put it somewhere else.
3. Add the broccoli florets to the same skillet and sauté for 4 to 5 minutes, or until they become tender but still retain some crispness.
4. In a small bowl, combine the soy sauce, water, cornstarch, honey, garlic, and ginger, and whisk them together. After adding the sauce to the broccoli in the pan, drizzle it evenly over the vegetables, and keep cooking for an additional 2 to 3 minutes, or until the sauce has thickened to the desired consistency.
5. Once the beef is fully cooked, return it to the skillet and stir it in with the other ingredients to combine. Allow the mixture to cook for an extra 2-3 minutes, or until it is heated through.
6. Divide the beef stir-fry between two plates and serve with brown rice or quinoa.

Nutritional Values (per serving):

Calories: 340 | Fat: 14g | Saturated Fat: 3g | Cholesterol: 80mg | Sodium: 820mg | Carbohydrates: 14g | Fiber: 2g | Sugar: 7g | Protein: 36g

BAKED CHICKEN FAJITA STUFFED PEPPERS

Ingredients:

- 2 large bell peppers, halved and seeded
- ½ lb boneless, skinless chicken breasts, cooked and shredded
- ¼ cup diced onion
- ¼ cup diced tomato
- ¼ cup low-sodium black beans, rinsed and drained
- ¼ cup frozen corn, thawed
- ¼ tsp chili powder
- ¼ tsp cumin
- ¼ tsp paprika
- ¼ tsp garlic powder
- ¼ tsp salt
- ¼ cup shredded reduced-fat cheddar cheese

Instructions:

1. Set the oven's temperature to 375°F (190°C). Line a baking sheet with parchment paper.
2. Combine the shredded chicken, onion, tomato, black beans, corn, cumin, paprika, garlic powder, and salt in a sizable bowl.
3. Stuff each bell pepper half with the chicken mixture, pressing firmly to fill the peppers.
4. Arrange the filled peppers onto the previously prepared baking sheet and cook them in the oven for about 25-30 minutes or until they have reached the desired tenderness.
5. Once the peppers are ready, remove them from the oven and sprinkle shredded cheddar cheese over them. To fully melt the cheese, place the dish back in the oven and reheat for another 2-3 minutes.
6. Once the stuffed peppers are ready, divide them evenly between two plates and serve.

Nutritional Values (per serving):

Calories: 290 | Fat: 6g | Saturated Fat: 2g | Cholesterol: 85mg | Sodium: 520mg | Carbohydrates: 23g | Fiber: 6g| Sugar: 7g | Protein: 36g

GREEK-STYLE GRILLED CHICKEN

Ingredients:

- 2 boneless, skinless chicken breasts
- ¼ cup plain low-fat Greek yogurt
- ¼ cup olive oil
- ¼ tsp garlic powder
- ¼ tsp dried oregano
- ¼ tsp dried thyme
- ¼ tsp salt
- ¼ tsp black pepper
- ½ lemon, juiced

Instructions:

1. In a shallow dish, mix together Greek yogurt, olive oil, garlic powder, dried oregano, dried thyme, salt, black pepper, and lemon juice.
2. Add the chicken breasts to the marinade, and turn them over to ensure they are fully coated. Cover the dish with a lid or plastic wrap, and refrigerate it for at least 30 minutes or up to 2 hours to allow it to chill and marinate.
3. Prior to grilling, preheat the grill or grill pan to high heat. Remove the chicken from the marinade, and shake off any excess marinade to ensure the chicken is not too wet.
4. The chicken should be cooked through, and the internal temperature reaches 165°F (74°C) by grilling it for 6-7 minutes on each side.
5. Before serving, take the chicken off the grill and allow it to rest for a brief period, usually a few minutes.

Nutritional Values (per serving):

Calories: 250 | Fat: 13g | Saturated Fat: 2g | Cholesterol: 85mg | Sodium: 380mg | Carbohydrates: 2g | Fiber: 0g | Sugar: 1g | Protein: 28g

BALSAMIC-GLAZED PORK CHOPS

Ingredients:

- 2 boneless pork chops, about 1/2 lb
- ¼ tsp salt
- ¼ tsp black pepper
- 1 tbsp olive oil
- ¼ cup balsamic vinegar
- 1 tbsp honey
- ¼ tsp dried rosemary

Instructions:

1. Add salt and black pepper to the pork chops.
2. In a pan, heat the olive oil over medium heat. Cook each side of the pork chops for only 4 to 5 minutes, as they should be fully cooked in this amount of time.
3. Whisk the balsamic vinegar, honey, and dried rosemary together in a small bowl.
4. The balsamic glaze should be applied to the pork chops after they have finished cooking. Cook the sauce for another 1 to 2 minutes, stirring it often, until it thickens and coats all of the pork chops.
5. After cooking, remove the pork chops from the pan and allow them to rest for a few minutes before serving.

Nutritional Values (per serving):

Calories: 280 | Fat: 14g | Saturated Fat: 3.5g | Cholesterol: 75mg | Sodium: 400mg | Carbohydrates: 10g | Fiber: 0g | Sugar: 9g | Protein: 28g

BEEF AND VEGETABLE STIR-FRY

Ingredients:

- ½ lb lean beef sirloin, thinly sliced
- ¼ tsp salt
- ¼ tsp black pepper
- 1 tbsp olive oil
- 1 cup mixed vegetables (such as bell peppers, carrots, and snap peas)
- ¼ cup low-sodium soy sauce
- ¼ cup water
- ½ tbsp cornstarch
- ½ tbsp honey
- ½ tsp minced garlic
- ½ tsp grated fresh ginger

Instructions:

1. Season the beef slices with salt and black pepper.
2. Using a large non-stick pan, heat the olive oil over medium heat. Add the beef to the pan and cook for 2-3 minutes on each side until it turns brown. Get the beef out of the pan and put it somewhere else.
3. Add the blend of vegetables to the skillet and cook for approximately 4 to 5 minutes until they are cooked enough to be tender yet retain their crispiness.
4. In a small bowl, combine and stir the soy sauce, water, cornstarch, honey, garlic, and ginger

thoroughly using a whisk. After whisking the sauce ingredients together, pour the mixture over the vegetables in the skillet. Cook for an additional 2 to 3 minutes or until the sauce has thickened to your desired consistency.
5. After cooking the beef, return it to the skillet along with the vegetables, and blend all ingredients together thoroughly to ensure they are well combined. Continue cooking the mixture for an additional 2-3 minutes, or until it is heated through and reaches the desired temperature.
6. Divide the beef and vegetable stir-fry between two plates and serve with brown rice or quinoa.

Nutritional Values (per serving):

Calories: 340 | Fat: 14g | Saturated Fat: 3g | Cholesterol: 80mg | Sodium: 820mg | Carbohydrates: 16g | Fiber: 3g | Sugar: 8g | Protein: 36g

SLOW COOKER BEEF STEW

Ingredients:

- ½ lb lean beef stew meat cubed
- ¼ tsp salt
- ¼ tsp black pepper
- ¼ tsp garlic powder
- ¼ tsp onion powder
- ¼ tsp paprika
- 1 tbsp olive oil
- 1 cup low-sodium beef broth
- ½ cup diced tomatoes
- 1 cup diced potatoes
- 1 cup sliced carrots
- 1 cup chopped celery
- ½ cup diced onion

Instructions:

1. Season the beef stew meat with salt, black pepper, garlic powder, onion powder, and paprika.
2. Heat up the olive oil in a nonstick skillet over medium heat until it becomes warm. Add the seasoned beef to the skillet and cook for around 4 to 5 minutes, or until it turns brown on all sides.
3. Move the browned beef from the skillet to a slow cooker using a spoon or spatula. Add the beef broth, diced tomatoes, diced potatoes, sliced carrots, chopped celery, and diced onion.
4. Set the slow cooker to low heat and let the beef and vegetables cook for approximately 7-8 hours, or alternatively, you can set it to high heat and cook for 4-5 hours until the beef is tender and the vegetables are thoroughly cooked.
5. Divide the beef stew between two bowls and serve.

Nutritional Values (per serving):

Calories: 350 | Fat: 12g | Saturated Fat: 3g | Cholesterol: 75mg | Sodium: 520mg | Carbohydrates: 27g | Fiber: 5g | Sugar: 6g | Protein: 30g

SHEET PAN SAUSAGE AND VEGETABLES

Ingredients:

- ½ lb turkey sausage, sliced
- 1 cup diced bell peppers
- 1 cup diced zucchini
- 1 cup diced red onion

- 1 cup cherry tomatoes
- 1 tbsp olive oil
- ¼ tsp salt
- ¼ tsp black pepper
- ¼ tsp garlic powder
- ¼ tsp dried basil
- ¼ tsp dried oregano

Instructions:

1. Set the oven's temperature to 400°F (200°C). Line a baking sheet with parchment paper.
2. In a large bowl, combine the sliced turkey sausage, diced bell peppers, diced zucchini, diced red onion, and cherry tomatoes. Add a drizzle of olive oil to the dish and sprinkle with salt, black pepper, garlic powder, dried basil, and dried oregano. Toss to coat.
3. Evenly distribute the sausage and vegetables on the prepared baking sheet, making sure they are spread out in a single layer.
4. Place the baking sheet in the oven and bake for approximately 20-25 minutes, or until the vegetables have softened, and the sausage has browned to the desired level.
5. Using a serving spoon, divide the sausage and vegetables equally between two plates and serve immediately.

Nutritional Values (per serving):

Calories: 320 | Fat: 16g | Saturated Fat: 3.5g | Cholesterol: 85mg | Sodium: 810mg | Carbohydrates: 19g | Fiber: 4g | Sugar: 9g | Protein: 26g

CHICKEN AND RICE STUFFED BELL PEPPERS

Ingredients:

- 2 large bell peppers, halved and seeded
- ½ lb boneless, skinless chicken breasts, cooked and shredded
- 1 cup cooked brown rice
- ¼ cup diced onion
- ¼ cup diced tomato
- ¼ cup low-sodium black beans, rinsed and drained
- ¼ cup frozen corn, thawed
- ¼ tsp salt
- ¼ tsp black pepper
- ¼ tsp cumin
- ¼ tsp paprika
- ¼ tsp garlic powder
- ¼ cup shredded reduced-fat cheddar cheese

Instructions:

1. Set the oven's temperature to 375°F (190°C). Line a baking sheet with parchment paper.
2. Combine the cooked brown rice, shredded chicken, onion, tomato, black beans, corn, salt, black pepper, cumin, garlic powder, and paprika in a large mixing bowl.
3. Stuff each bell pepper half with the chicken and rice mixture, pressing firmly to fill the peppers.
4. Arrange the stuffed peppers on the previously prepared baking sheet and bake them for around 25-30 minutes, or until the peppers have reached the desired level of tenderness.

5. Remove the peppers from the oven and evenly sprinkle shredded cheddar cheese over each pepper. Place the dish back in the oven and heat for an additional 2-3 minutes or until the cheese has completely melted.
6. Using a spatula or serving utensil, divide the stuffed peppers evenly between two plates and serve hot.

Nutritional Values (per serving):

Calories: 310 | Fat: 6g | Saturated Fat: 2g | Cholesterol: 85mg | Sodium: 540mg | Carbohydrates: 33g | Fiber: 6g | Sugar: 7g | Protein: 29g

SPAGHETTI SQUASH BOLOGNESE

Ingredients:

- 1 medium spaghetti squash, halved and seeded
- 1 tbsp olive oil
- ½ lb lean ground beef
- ¼ cup diced onion
- ¼ cup diced carrot
- ¼ cup diced celery
- ¼ tsp salt
- ¼ tsp black pepper
- 1 cup low-sodium marinara sauce
- ¼ cup grated Parmesan cheese

Instructions:

1. Set the oven's temperature to 400°F (200°C). Line a baking sheet with parchment paper.
2. Apply a layer of olive oil to the cut sides of the spaghetti squash and then put them face down on the baking sheet that has been prepared. Cook the squash for approximately 40-45 minutes or until it becomes tender enough to shred easily using a fork.
3. In the meantime, put a pan that doesn't stick on medium heat. Add the ground beef, diced onion, diced carrot, and diced celery—season with salt and black pepper. Using a spoon, break up the beef while cooking it with the vegetables for about 8-10 minutes, or until the beef turns brown, and the vegetables have become soft.
4. Add the marinara sauce to the skillet and stir well with the beef and vegetables. Cook the mixture for an additional 5 minutes, or until it is heated through and reaches the desired temperature.
5. Remove the spaghetti squash from the oven and let it cool down for a while before handling. Using a fork, scrape the inside of the squash to shred it into spaghetti-like strands.
6. Divide the spaghetti squash between two plates and top with the Bolognese beef sauce. Sprinkle with grated Parmesan cheese and serve.

Nutritional Values (per serving):

Calories: 420 | Fat: 21g | Saturated Fat: 7g | Cholesterol: 80mg | Sodium: 690mg | Carbohydrates: 32g | Fiber: 7g | Sugar: 13g | Protein: 27g

GARLIC HERB PORK TENDERLOIN

Ingredients:

- ½ lb pork tenderloin
- ¼ tsp salt
- ¼ tsp black pepper
- 1 tbsp olive oil
- 2 cloves garlic, minced
- ½ tsp dried rosemary
- ½ tsp dried thyme
- ½ tsp dried sage

Instructions:

1. Set the oven's temperature to 375°F (190°C). Line a baking sheet with parchment paper.
2. Season the pork tenderloin with salt and black pepper. Mix the minced garlic, dried rosemary, dried thyme, olive oil, and dried sage together in a small bowl.
3. Coat the entire pork tenderloin with the mixture, using your hands to press it down and help it stick to the meat.
4. Put the seasoned pork tenderloin on the prepared baking sheet and cook it in the oven for approximately 25-30 minutes or until it is thoroughly cooked.
5. Once the pork tenderloin is done cooking, remove it from the oven, and allow it to rest for a few minutes before slicing it.

Nutritional Values (per serving):

Calories: 250 | Fat: 14g | Saturated Fat: 3.5g | Cholesterol: 85mg | Sodium: 380mg | Carbohydrates: 1g | Fiber: 0g | Sugar: 0g | Protein: 27g

CHICKEN AND BROCCOLI STIR-FRY

Ingredients:

- ½ lb boneless, skinless chicken breasts, thinly sliced
- ¼ tsp salt
- ¼ tsp black pepper
- 1 tbsp olive oil
- 1 cup chopped broccoli
- ¼ cup low-sodium chicken broth
- ¼ cup low-sodium soy sauce
- ½ tbsp cornstarch
- ½ tbsp honey
- ½ tsp minced garlic
- ½ tsp grated fresh ginger

Instructions:

1. Season the chicken slices with salt and black pepper.
2. A big nonstick skillet should be heated with olive oil over medium heat. Add the chicken to the pan and cook each side for about 2 to 3 minutes or until the surface turns brown. Put the chicken on a plate. Take it out of the pan.
3. When the broccoli is soft but still has some crunch, add the chopped broccoli to the same pan and cook for an additional 4 to 5 minutes.
4. In a small bowl, combine the chicken broth, soy sauce, honey, garlic, and ginger. Mix the ingredients well. When the sauce has thickened, pour it over the broccoli and cook it for an additional 2 to 3 minutes. Put the cooked chicken back in the pan and stir it all together. Continue cooking the mixture for an additional 2-3 minutes, or until it is heated through and reaches the desired temperature.

5. Divide the chicken and broccoli stir-fry between two plates and serve with brown rice or quinoa.

Nutritional Values (per serving):

Calories: 300 | Fat: 10g | Saturated Fat: 1.5g | Cholesterol: 85mg | Sodium: 860mg | Carbohydrates: 16g | Fiber: 2g | Sugar: 8g | Protein: 34g

TURKEY MEATBALL SUBS

Ingredients:

- ½ lb lean ground turkey
- ¼ cup whole wheat breadcrumbs
- ¼ cup grated Parmesan cheese
- ¼ cup finely chopped fresh parsley
- ¼ tsp salt
- ¼ tsp black pepper
- ¼ tsp garlic powder
- 1 large egg, beaten
- 1 tbsp olive oil
- 1 cup low-sodium marinara sauce
- 2 whole wheat sub rolls, split
- ½ cup shredded reduced-fat mozzarella cheese

Instructions:

1. To start, in a sizable bowl, blend together the ground turkey, breadcrumbs, grated Parmesan cheese, chopped parsley, salt, black pepper, garlic powder, and beaten egg. Thoroughly combine and blend all the ingredients together until they are well mixed.
2. Shape the mixture into small meatballs, about 1-1.5 inches in diameter.
3. Heat the olive oil in a large non-stick pan over medium heat. Place the meatballs in the pan and cook for about 6-7 minutes, turning them occasionally, until they are browned on all sides.
4. Pour the marinara sauce over the meatballs in the skillet, making sure they are evenly coated, then cover the skillet with a lid. Lower the heat to a simmer and allow the mixture to cook for around 15-20 minutes or until the meatballs are fully cooked.
5. Preheat the broiler. Place the split sub rolls on a baking sheet.
6. Divide the meatballs and sauce evenly between the two sub rolls. Sprinkle shredded mozzarella cheese over the top of the meatballs and sauce in each sub roll.
7. Broil for two to three minutes or until the cheese is bubbly and melted. Remove from the oven and serve.

Nutritional Values (per serving):

Calories: 540 | Fat: 22g | Saturated Fat: 7g | Cholesterol: 130mg | Sodium: 980mg | Carbohydrates: 48g | Fiber: 6g | Sugar: 9g | Protein: 37g

GRILLED PORTOBELLO MUSHROOM BURGERS

Ingredients:

- 2 large portobello mushroom caps, cleaned and stems removed
- 1 tbsp olive oil
- ¼ tsp salt
- ¼ tsp black pepper
- ¼ tsp garlic powder
- ¼ tsp dried basil
- 2 whole wheat hamburger buns, split
- ½ cup sliced red onion
- ½ cup sliced tomato
- ¼ cup baby spinach leaves

Instructions:

1. Preheat the grill to medium-high heat.
2. Salt, black pepper, garlic powder, and dried basil are added to the portobello mushroom caps that have been brushed with olive oil.
3. Place the mushroom caps on the grill and cook for approximately 4-5 minutes per side, or until they are tender and have a slightly charred appearance.
4. Split the hamburger buns in half and toast them on the grill for 1 to 2 minutes until they are lightly browned.
5. To assemble the burgers, place a grilled portobello mushroom cap on the bottom half of each bun. Add sliced red onion, sliced tomato, and baby spinach leaves on top of the grilled portobello mushroom cap on each bun.

Nutritional Values (per serving):

Calories: 280 | Fat: 11g | Saturated Fat: 1.5g | Cholesterol: 0mg | Sodium: 500mg | Carbohydrates: 37g | Fiber: 6g | Sugar: 6g | Protein: 10g

GREEK CHICKEN PITA POCKETS

Ingredients:

- ½ lb boneless, skinless chicken breasts, thinly sliced
- ¼ tsp salt
- ¼ tsp black pepper
- ¼ tsp dried oregano
- 1 tbsp olive oil
- 2 whole wheat pita pockets, halved
- ½ cup chopped cucumber
- ½ cup chopped tomato
- ¼ cup sliced red onion
- ¼ cup crumbled feta cheese

Instructions:

1. Season the chicken slices with salt, black pepper, and dried oregano.
2. Heat up the olive oil in a non-stick pan over medium-high heat. Place the chicken in the pan and cook for 2 to 3 minutes per side, or until the chicken is fully cooked and browned. Put the chicken on a plate after removing it from the pan.
3. Warm the pita pockets for a few seconds in the oven or microwave to make them easier to work with.
4. Stuff each pita pocket half with cooked chicken, chopped cucumber, chopped tomato, sliced red onion, and crumbled feta cheese.

5. Serve the pita pockets with a side of Greek yogurt or tzatziki sauce for dipping, if desired.

Nutritional Values (per serving):

Calories: 380 | Fat: 12g | Saturated Fat: 4g | Cholesterol: 85mg | Sodium: 720mg | Carbohydrates: 38g | Fiber: 6g | Sugar: 4g | Protein: 31g

PHILLY CHEESESTEAK STUFFED PEPPERS

Ingredients:

- 2 large green bell peppers, halved and seeded
- ½ lb lean beef sirloin, thinly sliced
- ¼ tsp salt
- ¼ tsp black pepper
- 1 tbsp olive oil
- ½ cup sliced onion
- ½ cup sliced mushrooms
- ¼ cup shredded reduced-fat provolone cheese

Instructions:

1. Set the oven's temperature to 375°F (190°C). Cover a baking sheet with parchment paper.
2. Sprinkle salt and black pepper over the beef sirloin slices to season them.
3. Heat the olive oil in a non-stick pan over medium heat. Put the beef, onion, and mushrooms in the pan. Cook the beef and vegetables for 4-5 minutes, occasionally stirring until the beef is browned and the vegetables are tender.
4. Stuff the beef and vegetable mixture into each half of the bell pepper. Shred some provolone cheese and put it on top.
5. On the baking sheet previously prepared, bake the stuffed peppers for around 20-25 minutes until the cheese has melted and is bubbly.
6. Divide the Philly cheesesteak stuffed peppers between two plates and serve.

Nutritional Values (per serving):

Calories: 330 | Fat: 15g | Saturated Fat: 5g | Cholesterol: 75mg | Sodium: 590mg | Carbohydrates: 14g | Fiber: 3g | Sugar: 6g | Protein: 33g

BBQ-PULLED CHICKEN SANDWICHES

Ingredients:

- ½ lb boneless, skinless chicken breasts
- ¼ tsp salt
- ¼ tsp black pepper
- ½ cup low-sodium chicken broth
- ½ cup BBQ sauce, divided
- 2 whole wheat hamburger buns, split
- ½ cup coleslaw

Instructions:

1. Season the chicken breasts with a sprinkle of salt and black pepper.
2. Add the chicken, chicken broth, and 1/4 cup of BBQ sauce to a

slow cooker. Slow-cook the chicken for 4-5 hours on low or 2-3 hours on high until it is fully cooked and can be effortlessly shredded with a fork.
3. After removing the chicken from the slow cooker, use two forks to shred the chicken apart. Stir in the remaining 1/4 cup of BBQ sauce, making sure it is evenly distributed throughout the shredded chicken.
4. Divide the shredded BBQ chicken between the two split hamburger buns. Top each sandwich with coleslaw and serve.

Nutritional Values (per serving):

Calories: 380 | Fat: 6g | Saturated Fat: 1g | Cholesterol: 80mg | Sodium: 810mg | Carbohydrates: 46g | Fiber: 4g | Sugar: 19g | Protein: 34g

BEEF AND VEGETABLE-STIR FRY

Ingredients:

- ½ lb lean beef sirloin, thinly sliced
- ¼ tsp salt
- ¼ tsp black pepper
- 1 tbsp olive oil
- 1 cup chopped bell peppers (any color)
- 1 cup chopped zucchini
- ¼ cup low-sodium beef broth
- ¼ cup low-sodium soy sauce
- ½ tbsp cornstarch
- ½ tbsp honey
- ½ tsp minced garlic
- ½ tsp grated fresh ginger

Instructions:

1. Season the beef slices with salt and black pepper.
2. Heat up the olive oil in a large non-stick pan over medium heat. Add the beef to the pan and cook for approximately 2 to 3 minutes per side, or until it is browned. Take the beef out of the skillet and put it somewhere else.
3. Incorporate the bell peppers and zucchini into the same pan. Continue cooking the beef and vegetables for about 4 to 5 minutes, or until the vegetables have softened but still retain some crunchiness
4. In a small mixing bowl, whisk together the beef stock, soy sauce, cornstarch, honey, garlic, and ginger until they are thoroughly combined. Add the mixture from the small mixing bowl to the pan with the vegetables and beef. Continue cooking the mixture for another 2 to 3 minutes or until the sauce thickens to the desired consistency.
5. Return the cooked beef to the skillet, and stir it together with the vegetables and sauce until they are thoroughly combined. Continue cooking the mixture for an additional 2-3 minutes, or until it is heated through and reaches the desired temperature.
6. Divide the beef and vegetable stir-fry between two plates and serve with brown rice or quinoa.

Nutritional Values (per serving):

Calories: 330 | Fat: 12g | Saturated Fat: 2.5g | Cholesterol: 60mg | Sodium: 860mg | Carbohydrates: 19g | Fiber: 2g | Sugar: 9g | Protein: 33g

TURKEY TACO WRAPS

Ingredients:

- ½ lb lean ground turkey
- ¼ tsp salt
- ¼ tsp black pepper
- ¼ tsp cumin
- ¼ tsp paprika
- ¼ tsp garlic powder
- ¼ cup low-sodium chicken broth
- 6 large iceberg or butter lettuce leaves
- ½ cup chopped tomato
- ¼ cup shredded reduced-fat cheddar cheese
- ¼ cup salsa

Instructions:

1. The ground turkey should be cooked in a nonstick skillet over medium heat while being broken up with a spoon. Add salt, black pepper, cumin, paprika, and garlic powder to taste. Cook until browned and fully cooked through.
2. Add the chicken broth to the pan and cook the mixture for an additional 2-3 minutes, or until the liquid has evaporated and the ingredients are well combined.
3. Incorporate the turkey mixture into lettuce leaves. Top with chopped tomato, shredded cheddar cheese, and salsa.
4. Take the lettuce leaves and use them to wrap around the filling, ensuring that the filling is completely covered by the lettuce. Serve the dish immediately.

Nutritional Values (per serving):

Calories: 230 | Fat: 9g | Saturated Fat: 3g | Cholesterol: 80mg | Sodium: 690mg | Carbohydrates: 9g | Fiber: 2g | Sugar: 4g | Protein: 27g

BALSAMIC GLAZED CHICKEN

Ingredients:

- ½ lb boneless, skinless chicken breasts
- ¼ tsp salt
- ¼ tsp black pepper
- 1 tbsp olive oil
- ¼ cup balsamic vinegar
- ½ tbsp honey
- ½ tbsp Dijon mustard
- ½ tsp minced garlic
- ¼ tsp dried rosemary

Instructions:

1. Add salt and black pepper to the chicken breasts.
2. Heat up the olive oil in a nonstick pan over medium heat.
3. Add the chicken breasts and cook for 5–6 minutes per side or until they are fully cooked and browned.
4. Mix the balsamic vinegar, honey, Dijon mustard, minced garlic, and dried rosemary in a small bowl with a whisk.
5. Pour the glaze made from balsamic vinegar over the chicken breasts in the pan. Cook the

chicken for 2-3 minutes on low heat until the glaze thickens and evenly coats the chicken.
6. Remove the chicken from the pan before cutting it into desired pieces.
7. Divide the chicken with balsamic glaze between two plates and serve with any side dishes you like.

Nutritional Values (per serving):

Calories: 270 | Fat: 10g | Saturated Fat: 2g | Cholesterol: 80mg | Sodium: 560mg | Carbohydrates: 14g | Fiber: 0g | Sugar: 12g | Protein: 30g

SAUSAGE, PEPPERS, AND ONIONS SKILLETS

Ingredients:

- ½ lb Italian turkey sausage, sliced
- 1 tbsp olive oil
- 1 cup sliced bell peppers (any color)
- 1 cup sliced onion
- ¼ cup low-sodium chicken broth
- ¼ cup low-sodium marinara sauce
- ¼ tsp dried oregano
- ¼ tsp dried basil

Instructions:

1. In a big nonstick skillet, warm the olive oil over medium heat. Add the sliced turkey sausage to the pan and cook for 4-5 minutes, turning the slices occasionally until they are browned on all sides. From the skillet, take out the sausage, and set it aside.
2. In the same pan, combine the bell peppers and onions. Cook the vegetables for 5 to 6 minutes while occasionally stirring until they are soft.
3. Return the cooked sausage to the skillet. Stir in the chicken broth, marinara sauce, dried oregano, and dried basil. Continue cooking the mixture for an additional 3-4 minutes, or until it is heated through and reaches the desired temperature.
4. Divide the sausage, peppers, and onions skillet between two plates and serve.

Nutritional Values (per serving):

Calories: 340 | Fat: 19g | Saturated Fat: 4g | Cholesterol: 70mg | Sodium: 930mg | Carbohydrates: 20g | Fiber: 4g | Sugar: 9g | Protein: 24g

ROSEMARY LEMON PORK CHOPS

Ingredients:

- ½ lb boneless pork chops (about 2 chops)
- ¼ tsp salt
- ¼ tsp black pepper
- 1 tbsp olive oil
- ¼ cup lemon juice
- ¼ cup low-sodium chicken broth
- ½ tsp minced garlic
- ½ tsp dried rosemary

Instructions:

1. Add salt and black pepper to the pork chops.
2. Heat up the olive oil in a non-stick pan over medium heat. Once the pork chops have been added to the pan, cook them for approximately 4-5 minutes on each side.
3. Using a whisk, combine the lemon juice, chicken broth, minced garlic, and dried rosemary in a small bowl until they are well mixed. Pour the mixture over the pork chops in the pan.
4. Keep cooking the sauce on low heat for another three to four minutes or until it starts to get a little thicker.
5. Divide the rosemary lemon pork chops between two plates and serve with your choice of side dishes.

Nutritional Values (per serving):

Calories: 300 | Fat: 18g | Saturated Fat: 4g | Cholesterol: 90mg | Sodium: 430mg | Carbohydrates: 3g | Fiber: 0g | Sugar: 1g | Protein: 29g

MOROCCAN-SPICED BEEF STEW

Ingredients:

- ½ lb lean beef stew meat
- ¼ tsp salt
- ¼ tsp black pepper
- 1 tbsp olive oil
- ½ cup chopped onion
- ½ cup chopped carrot
- ½ cup chopped celery
- ½ cup low-sodium beef broth
- ½ cup canned diced tomatoes, undrained
- ½ tsp ground cumin
- ½ tsp ground coriander
- ¼ tsp ground cinnamon
- ¼ tsp paprika
- ¼ cup chopped fresh cilantro

Instructions:

1. Add salt and black pepper to the beef stew meat.
2. Heat the olive oil over medium heat in a large pot or Dutch oven. Add the beef and cook it, turning it occasionally, for 4–5 minutes or until all sides are browned. Take the beef out of the pot and set it aside on a plate or bowl.
3. Add the onion, carrot, and celery to the same pot. Cook for 4-5 minutes, occasionally stirring, until the vegetables are softened.
4. Return the cooked beef to the pot. Stir in the beef broth, diced tomatoes, ground cumin, ground coriander, ground cinnamon, and paprika. Bring the mixture to a boil.
5. Once the beef is tender and the flavors are well-balanced, reduce the heat to low, cover the pot, and let it simmer for an hour to an hour and a half.
6. Add the chopped fresh cilantro to the pot just before serving and stir it in well to ensure it is evenly distributed throughout the dish. Divide the Moroccan-spiced beef stew between two bowls and serve.

Nutritional Values (per serving):

Calories: 350 | Fat: 16g | Saturated Fat: 4g | Cholesterol: 85mg | Sodium: 540mg | Carbohydrates: 17g | Fiber: 4g | Sugar: 6g | Protein: 34g

SPINACH AND FETA STUFFED CHICKEN BREASTS

Ingredients:

- 2 boneless, skinless chicken breasts
- ¼ tsp salt
- ¼ tsp black pepper
- ½ cup chopped fresh spinach
- ¼ cup crumbled feta cheese
- 1 tbsp olive oil
- ¼ cup low-sodium chicken broth

Instructions:

1. Set the oven's temperature to 375°F (190°C).
2. Using a sharp knife, carefully cut a horizontal pocket into each chicken breast without slicing it all the way through.
3. Season the chicken breasts with salt and black pepper to taste.
4. Put half of the chopped spinach and crumbled feta cheese in each chicken breast pocket.
5. Place a large oven-safe skillet on medium heat and heat up the olive oil until it's hot.
6. Add the chicken breasts that have been stuffed with stuffing and cook them for 4 to 5 minutes on each side until they are browned.
7. Place the pan in an already-heated oven after adding the chicken broth to it. Bake the chicken for approximately 15 to 20 minutes or until it is completely cooked through.
8. Divide the spinach and feta stuffed chicken breasts between two plates and serve with your choice of side dishes.

Nutritional Values (per serving):

Calories: 300 | Fat: 15g | Saturated Fat: 4g | Cholesterol: 100mg | Sodium: 620mg | Carbohydrates: 2g | Fiber: 1g | Sugar: 1g | Protein: 36g

ASIAN TURKEY LETTUCE WRAPS

Ingredients:

- ½ lb lean ground turkey
- ¼ cup hoisin sauce
- 1 tbsp low-sodium soy sauce
- ½ tbsp rice vinegar
- ½ tbsp grated fresh ginger
- ½ tbsp minced garlic
- ½ cup chopped water chestnuts
- ¼ cup chopped green onions
- ¼ cup chopped fresh cilantro
- 6 large iceberg or butter lettuce leaves
- Optional toppings: chopped peanuts, Sriracha sauce

Instructions:

1. Spoon-break ground turkey in a non-stick skillet over medium heat. Cook until browned and fully cooked through.
2. Mix hoisin sauce, soy sauce, rice vinegar, grated ginger, and

minced garlic in a small bowl. After the turkey is cooked, pour the sauce over it and stir until the sauce is evenly distributed and fully combined with the turkey.

3. Add the chopped water chestnuts, green onions, and fresh cilantro to the skillet and stir them in until they are well combined with the other ingredients. Cook the combined ingredients for an additional 2-3 minutes until they are heated through and ready to be served.
4. Using a spoon, place the ground turkey mixture into the lettuce leaves. Add optional toppings such as chopped peanuts or Sriracha sauce, if desired.
5. Take lettuce leaves and fold them around the filling, making sure to wrap them securely. Serve immediately.

Nutritional Values (per serving):

Calories: 230 | Fat: 7g | Saturated Fat: 2g | Cholesterol: 60mg | Sodium: 860mg | Carbohydrates: 20g | Fiber: 3g | Sugar: 9g | Protein: 22g

SEAFOODS RECIPE

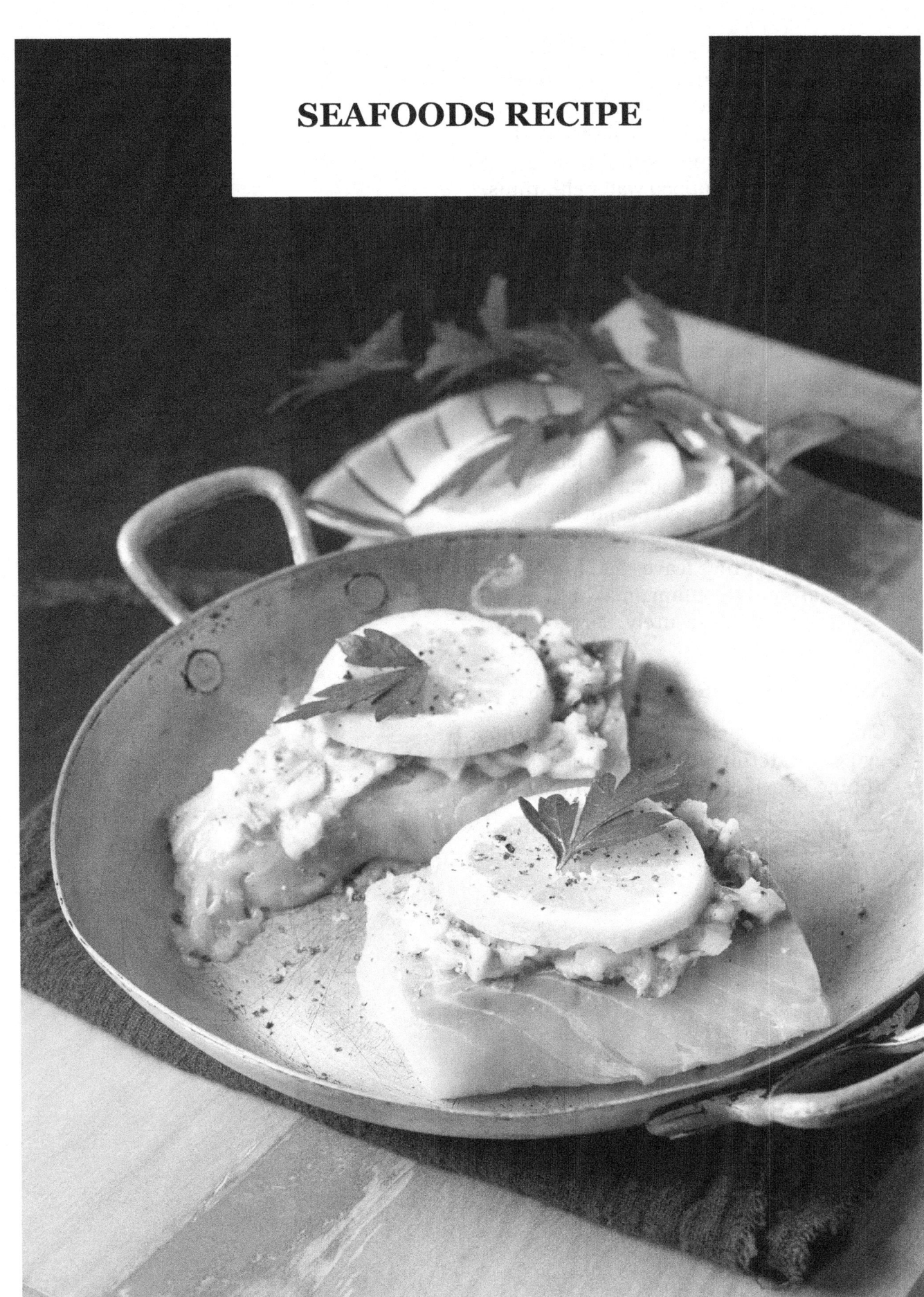

LEMON GARLIC BAKED COD

Ingredients:

- 2 (6 oz) cod fillets
- 2 tbsp olive oil
- 2 cloves garlic, minced
- ½ lemon, juiced
- ¼ tsp salt
- ¼ tsp black pepper
- 1 tbsp chopped fresh parsley

Instructions:

1. Set the oven's temperature to 400°F (200°C). Take a baking sheet and cover it with parchment paper to prevent the food from sticking to the surface of the sheet.
2. Combine olive oil, minced garlic, lemon juice, salt, and black pepper in a small bowl and whisk all the ingredients together until they are fully blended.
3. Put the cod fillets on the baking sheet that has been prepared and brush them with the lemon-garlic mixture.
4. Cook the fish in the oven for a duration of 12 to 15 minutes or until it becomes tender enough to break apart effortlessly using a fork.
5. Garnish with chopped fresh parsley and serve.

Nutritional Values (per serving):

Calories: 210 | Fat: 11g | Saturated Fat: 1.5g | Cholesterol: 65mg | Sodium: 390mg | Carbohydrates: 2g | Fiber: 0g | Sugar: 0g | Protein: 24g

SHRIMP AND VEGGIE STIR-FRY

Ingredients:

- 1 tbsp olive oil
- ½ lb raw shrimp, peeled and deveined
- ½ cup sliced bell pepper
- ½ cup sliced onion
- ½ cup snow peas
- ½ cup broccoli florets
- 1 tbsp low-sodium soy sauce
- 1 tbsp oyster sauce
- ½ tbsp honey
- ½ tbsp cornstarch
- ¼ cup water

Instructions:

1. Start by warming up the olive oil in a generously sized frying pan or wok, using medium-high heat.
2. Once the oil has attained the desired temperature, place the shrimp into the frying pan and cook for approximately 2-3 minutes on each side until it transforms into a pleasing pink color and is fully cooked. After cooking, take the shrimp out of the skillet and put it aside for later use.
3. Add bell pepper, onion, snow peas, and broccoli in the same skillet. Cook the vegetables for 4-5 minutes, stirring occasionally, until they are tender and cooked to your liking.
4. In a small bowl, whisk together soy sauce, oyster sauce, honey, cornstarch, and water until the mixture is well blended.

5. Add the cooked shrimp back to the pan and stir everything together until the sauce is evenly distributed and all the ingredients are well combined. Cook the mixture for an additional 2-3 minutes or until the sauce thickens to your desired consistency. Keep stirring occasionally to ensure that the sauce does not burn or stick to the pan.
6. Divide the shrimp and veggie stir-fry between two plates and serve.

Nutritional Values (per serving):

Calories: 280 | Fat: 10g | Saturated Fat: 1.5g | Cholesterol: 170mg | Sodium: 840mg | Carbohydrates: 21g | Fiber: 3g | Sugar: 9g | Protein: 26g

PAN-SEARED SCALLOPS WITH GARLIC SPINACH

Ingredients:

- 6 large sea scallops, patted dry
- 1 tbsp olive oil
- 1 tbsp unsalted butter
- 1 clove garlic, minced
- 4 cups fresh spinach
- ¼ tsp salt
- ¼ tsp black pepper
- ¼ tsp crushed red pepper flakes (optional)

Instructions:

1. In a large pan, heat a half tablespoon of olive oil over medium-high heat.
2. Season the scallops with salt and black pepper to taste. Place the scallops in the heated pan and cook for approximately 2-3 minutes on both sides until they are evenly cooked and achieve a golden-brown color. Once done, transfer the scallops from the pan onto a plate.
3. Using the same pan, heat the remaining half tablespoon of olive oil and the butter until the butter is fully melted and the oil is hot. Place the diced garlic into the pan and sauté for about a minute or until a pleasant aroma emanates from the garlic.
4. Add fresh spinach, salt, black pepper, and crushed red pepper flakes (if using) to the pan and stir everything together until the spinach wilts and becomes tender.
5. Divide the garlic spinach evenly between two plates, place the cooked scallops on top of the spinach, and serve immediately.

Nutritional Values (per serving):

Calories: 260 | Fat: 17g | Saturated Fat: 5g | Cholesterol: 45mg | Sodium: 700mg | Carbohydrates: 6g | Fiber: 2g | Sugar: 1g | Protein: 20g

SALMON WITH DILL YOGURT SAUCE

Ingredients:

- 2 (4 oz) salmon fillets
- ½ tsp salt
- ¼ tsp black pepper
- ½ cup plain Greek yogurt
- 1 tbsp chopped fresh dill

- 1 tsp lemon juice
- ½ tsp garlic powder

Instructions:

1. Set the oven to 425°F (220°C) and turn it on. Put parchment paper on a baking sheet.
2. Add salt and black pepper to the salmon filets. Arrange them on the baking sheet with the skin side facing down.
3. Allow the salmon to bake for a duration of 12-15 minutes or until it is thoroughly cooked and can be effortlessly flaked apart using a fork.
4. In a small bowl, mix together fresh dill, garlic powder, lemon juice, and Greek yogurt until the ingredients are well combined.
5. Serve the cooked salmon with a dollop of dill yogurt sauce.

Nutritional Values (per serving):

Calories: 300 | Fat: 15g | Saturated Fat: 3g | Cholesterol: 80mg | Sodium: 720mg | Carbohydrates: 3g | Fiber: 0g | Sugar: 2g | Protein: 35g

CRAB CAKES WITH LEMON AIOLI

Ingredients:

For the crab cakes:

- 8 oz lump crabmeat, drained
- ¼ cup whole wheat breadcrumbs
- ¼ cup chopped fresh parsley
- ¼ cup chopped green onions
- ¼ cup mayonnaise
- ¼ tsp salt
- ¼ tsp black pepper
- 1 large egg, lightly beaten
- 2 tbsp olive oil

For the lemon aioli:

- ¼ cup mayonnaise
- 1 tbsp lemon juice
- 1 tsp grated lemon zest
- ¼ tsp garlic powder

Instructions:

1. In a large bowl, combine the crabmeat, breadcrumbs, parsley, green onions, mayonnaise, salt, black pepper, and beaten egg. Gently mix until well combined.
2. Make crab cakes from each of the four equal parts of the mixture.
3. To prepare the crab cakes, it is recommended to heat a nonstick skillet over medium heat and add olive oil to the skillet. After heating the skillet, the crab cakes should be cooked for around 3-4 minutes on each side until they achieve a consistent, golden brown color and are uniformly heated throughout.
4. Combine all the ingredients for the lemon aioli in a small bowl and mix them together thoroughly.
5. Add a dollop of lemon aioli to the crab cakes and serve.

Nutritional Values (per serving):

Calories: 420 | Fat: 32g | Saturated Fat: 4.5g | Cholesterol: 135mg | Sodium:

980mg | Carbohydrates: 10g | Fiber: 1g | Sugar: 2g | Protein: 20g

ONE-PAN SHRIMP AND ASPARAGUS

Ingredients:

- ½ lb raw shrimp, peeled and deveined
- ½ lb asparagus, trimmed
- 1 tbsp olive oil
- ½ lemon, juiced
- 2 cloves garlic, minced
- ¼ tsp salt
- ¼ tsp black pepper
- ¼ tsp crushed red pepper flakes (optional)

Instructions:

1. To start, you should preheat your oven to 400°F (200°C). Following this, prepare your baking sheet by covering it with parchment paper.
2. Combine the prawns, asparagus, olive oil, lemon juice, garlic, salt, black pepper, and optional crushed red pepper flakes (if desired) in a spacious bowl, and mix thoroughly. Spread the shrimp and asparagus mixture evenly on the prepared baking sheet.
3. Cook the shrimp and asparagus for a duration of 10-12 minutes, or until the shrimp have turned pink and are fully cooked while the asparagus has reached a state of tenderness.
4. Divide the one-pan shrimp and asparagus between two plates and serve.

Nutritional Values (per serving):

Calories: 190 | Fat: 8g | Saturated Fat: 1g | Cholesterol: 145mg | Sodium: 720mg | Carbohydrates: 9g | Fiber: 3g | Sugar: 3g | Protein: 22g

BAKED TILAPIA WITH MEDITERRANEAN SALSA

Ingredients:

- 2 (6 oz) tilapia fillets
- ½ cup chopped tomatoes
- ¼ cup chopped cucumber
- ¼ cup chopped red onion
- ¼ cup chopped Kalamata olives
- ¼ cup chopped fresh parsley
- 1 tbsp olive oil
- ½ lemon, juiced
- ¼ tsp salt
- ¼ tsp black pepper

Instructions:

1. To start, you should preheat your oven to 400°F (200°C). Following this, prepare your baking sheet by covering it with parchment paper.
2. Season the tilapia fillets with salt and black pepper to taste. Then place them on the prepared baking sheet.
3. Cook the fish in the oven for approximately 12 to 15 minutes or until it becomes tender enough to be separated easily with a fork.
4. In a medium bowl, mix together the tomatoes, cucumber, red onion, Kalamata olives, parsley, olive oil, and lemon juice until all the ingredients are well combined.

5. Serve the cooked tilapia topped with Mediterranean salsa.

Nutritional Values (per serving):

Calories: 300 | Fat: 13g | Saturated Fat: 2g | Cholesterol: 85mg | Sodium: 700mg | Carbohydrates: 9g | Fiber: 2g | Sugar: 4g | Protein: 36g

EASY CLAM SPAGHETTI

Ingredients:

- 4 oz whole wheat spaghetti
- 1 tbsp olive oil
- ¼ cup chopped onion
- 2 cloves garlic, minced
- 1 (6.5 oz) can of chopped clams, drained (reserve the juice)
- ¼ cup clam juice (from the can)
- ¼ cup chopped fresh parsley
- ¼ tsp crushed red pepper flakes (optional)
- ¼ tsp black pepper

Instructions:

1. Cook the whole wheat spaghetti according to package instructions until al dente. Drain the mixture and set it aside.
2. Heat the olive oil in a large skillet over medium heat. Afterward, include the onion and garlic, and let it cook for approximately 3-4 minutes until the onion turns translucent.
3. Introduce the chopped clams, clam juice, parsley, black pepper, and optionally crushed red pepper flakes into the skillet. Cook for 5 minutes, stirring occasionally.
4. Toss the cooked spaghetti with the clam sauce. Divide the spaghetti evenly between two plates and serve immediately.

Nutritional Values (per serving):

Calories: 350 | Fat: 9g | Saturated Fat: 1g | Cholesterol: 20mg | Sodium: 570mg | Carbohydrates: 50g | Fiber: 6g | Sugar: 2g | Protein: 20g

SEARED AHI TUNA WITH MANGO SALSA

Ingredients:

- 2 (4 oz) ahi tuna steaks
- ½ tsp salt
- ¼ tsp black pepper
- 1 tbsp olive oil

For the mango salsa:

- ½ cup diced mango
- ¼ cup diced red bell pepper
- ¼ cup chopped red onion
- ¼ cup chopped fresh cilantro
- ½ jalapeño, seeded and minced
- ½ lime, juiced
- ¼ tsp salt

Instructions:

1. Pat the ahi tuna steaks dry with paper towels and season them with salt and black pepper.
2. Warm up the olive oil using a non-stick pan on medium to high heat. Add the tuna steaks to the pan and sear them on each side for 1-2 minutes, or until the outer

layer is seared and the center is still pink.
3. For the mango salsa, combine freshly diced mango, finely chopped red bell pepper, and red onion in a medium-sized bowl. Add in the minced jalapeño, fresh cilantro, lime juice, and salt. Mix all the ingredients together thoroughly.
4. Serve the seared ahi tuna topped with mango salsa.

Nutritional Values (per serving):

Calories: 270 | Fat: 11g | Saturated Fat: 2g | Cholesterol: 45mg | Sodium: 810mg | Carbohydrates: 13g | Fiber: 2g | Sugar: 10g | Protein: 30g

SEAFOOD PAELLA

Ingredients:

- 1 tbsp olive oil
- ¼ cup chopped onion
- ¼ cup chopped red bell pepper
- ¼ cup chopped green bell pepper
- ½ cup Arborio rice
- 1 cup low-sodium chicken or vegetable broth
- ¼ tsp saffron threads
- ¼ tsp paprika
- ¼ tsp salt
- ¼ tsp black pepper
- ½ cup canned diced tomatoes drained
- ½ cup frozen peas, thawed
- ½ lb mixed seafood (shrimp, scallops, mussels, and/or squid)
- ¼ cup chopped fresh parsley

Instructions:

1. Begin by warming up the olive oil in a generously-sized skillet set to medium heat.
2. Toss in the diced onion, red bell pepper, and green bell pepper, and allow the mixture to cook for around 4 to 5 minutes or until the vegetables have softened to your liking.
3. Add the Arborio rice to the skillet, stirring to coat the rice with oil. Cook for 2 minutes, stirring occasionally.
4. Stir in the chicken or vegetable broth, saffron threads, paprika, salt, black pepper, and diced tomatoes. Bring the combination to a boiling point, then reduce the temperature and allow it to simmer for 15 minutes, stirring occasionally.
5. Add the peas and mixed seafood to the skillet. After covering the dish, allow it to cook for an additional 10-15 minutes until the rice has softened and the seafood has been fully cooked.
6. Lastly, add the chopped fresh parsley and serve.

Nutritional Values (per serving):

Calories: 390 | Fat: 9g | Saturated Fat: 1.5g | Cholesterol: 120mg | Sodium: 710mg | Carbohydrates: 52g | Fiber: 4g | Sugar: 5g | Protein: 26g

BAKED COD WITH CHERRY TOMATOES AND OLIVES

Ingredients:

- 2 (6 oz) cod fillets
- ½ cup cherry tomatoes, halved

- ¼ cup pitted Kalamata olives, halved
- 1 tbsp olive oil
- ½ lemon, juiced
- ¼ tsp salt
- ¼ tsp black pepper
- ¼ cup chopped fresh basil

Instructions:

1. Warm up the oven to a temperature of 400°F (200°C). Put parchment paper on a baking sheet.
2. Prepare the baking sheet in advance and arrange the cod fillets on it. To enhance their flavor, sprinkle a pinch of black pepper and salt over them
3. Combine the cherry tomatoes, Kalamata olives, olive oil, and lemon juice in a medium bowl. Mix well.
4. Distribute the mixture of tomatoes and olives on top of the cod fillets.
5. Put the prepared dish inside the oven and cook for roughly 12 to 15 minutes or until the fish can be easily separated with a fork.
6. Garnish with chopped fresh basil and serve.

Nutritional Values (per serving):

Calories: 240 | Fat: 10g | Saturated Fat: 1.5g | Cholesterol: 65mg | Sodium: 670mg | Carbohydrates: 6g | Fiber: 1g | Sugar: 3g | Protein: 30g

GARLIC BUTTER SCALLOPS

Ingredients:

- 8 large sea scallops, patted dry
- 1 tbsp olive oil
- 2 tbsp unsalted butter
- 2 cloves garlic, minced
- ¼ tsp salt
- ¼ tsp black pepper
- ¼ cup chopped fresh parsley
- ½ lemon, juiced

Instructions:

1. Heat up the olive oil in a large non-stick pan over medium heat.
2. Once the oil has reached the ideal temperature, carefully add the scallops to the pan and cook for approximately 2 to 3 minutes on each side until they are fully cooked and have turned a crisp golden brown. Place the scallops on a plate after removing them from the pan.
3. Melt the butter in the skillet over medium heat until it is fully melted.
4. Once melted, introduce the garlic and let it cook for around 1 to 2 minutes until you can smell its aroma.
5. Add the scallops back to the skillet with the melted butter and season them with salt and black pepper to taste. Cook the scallops for an additional 1-2 minutes until they are heated through and fully cooked. Keep stirring them gently to ensure that they are evenly cooked on all sides.
6. After cooking the scallops, stir in the chopped parsley and lemon juice until all the ingredients are well combined. Divide the garlic

butter scallops between two plates and serve.

Nutritional Values (per serving):

Calories: 240 | Fat: 16g | Saturated Fat: 6g | Cholesterol: 65mg| Sodium: 540mg | Carbohydrates: 6g | Fiber: 0g | Sugar: 0g | Protein: 20g

LEMON HERB BAKED SALMON

Ingredients:

- 2 (6 oz) salmon fillets
- 1 tbsp olive oil
- ½ lemon, juiced
- ¼ tsp salt
- ¼ tsp black pepper
- ¼ tsp dried thyme
- ¼ tsp dried rosemary
- ¼ tsp dried oregano
- ½ lemon, sliced

Instructions:

1. To begin, preheat your oven to 375°F (190°C) and then prepare a baking sheet by lining it with parchment paper. This will prevent the food from sticking to the sheet during the cooking process.
2. Arrange the salmon fillets onto the prepared baking sheet, making sure to leave some space between each fillet. This will ensure that they cook evenly and thoroughly. Sprinkle with salt, black pepper, thyme, rosemary, and oregano, and then drizzle with olive oil and lemon juice.
3. Place the lemon slices on top of the salmon fillets.
4. Cook the salmon in the oven for a duration of 12 to 15 minutes or until it reaches a point where it can be easily separated with a fork.
5. Divide the lemon herb baked salmon between two plates and serve.

Nutritional Values (per serving):

Calories: 300 | Fat: 18g | Saturated Fat: 3g | Cholesterol: 85mg | Sodium: 370mg | Carbohydrates: 2g | Fiber: 1g | Sugar: 0g | Protein: 31g

SPICY CAJUN SHRIMP SKILLET

Ingredients:

- 1 tbsp olive oil
- ½ lb shrimp, peeled and deveined
- ¼ cup chopped onion
- ¼ cup chopped bell pepper
- ¼ cup chopped celery
- ¼ cup low-sodium vegetable broth
- ¼ cup canned diced tomatoes
- ¼ tsp cajun seasoning
- ¼ tsp salt
- ¼ tsp black pepper
- ¼ cup chopped green onions

Instructions:

1. To initiate the cooking process, warm up the olive oil in a generously proportioned skillet or wok over medium-high heat.

2. After the oil has been heated, add the shrimp and cook it for approximately 2-3 minutes on both sides until it attains a delightful shade of pink and is cooked thoroughly. After cooking, take the shrimp out of the skillet and put it aside for later use.
3. In the same skillet, add the onion, bell pepper, and celery. Cook the vegetables for 4-5 minutes or until they have softened to your desired consistency.
4. Stir in the vegetable broth, diced tomatoes, Cajun seasoning, salt, and black pepper. Heat the mixture over low-medium heat for approximately 5-6 minutes, occasionally stirring until the sauce reaches a slightly thicker consistency. After that, transfer the shrimp back into the skillet and continue cooking for an extra 1-2 minutes until they are completely heated through.
5. Stir in the chopped green onions. Divide the spicy Cajun shrimp skillet between two plates and serve.

Nutritional Values (per serving):

Calories: 230 | Fat: 9g | Saturated Fat: 1.5g | Cholesterol: 180mg | Sodium: 630mg | Carbohydrates: 9g | Fiber: 2g | Sugar: 4g | Protein: 29g

MISO-GLAZED SALMON

Ingredients:

- 2 (6 oz) salmon fillets
- 1 tbsp white miso paste
- 1 tbsp mirin
- 1 tbsp low-sodium soy sauce
- ½ tsp sesame oil
- ½ tsp honey
- ½ tsp grated ginger

Instructions:

1. Warm up the oven to a temperature of 400°F (200°C). Put parchment paper on a baking sheet.
2. Whisk the miso paste, mirin, soy sauce, sesame oil, honey, and grated ginger together in a small bowl.
3. Lay the salmon fillets on the prepared baking sheet and brush them with the miso mixture.
4. Arrange the salmon on a baking sheet and place it in the oven, baking for approximately 10-12 minutes or until it becomes flaky and can be easily separated with a fork.
5. Divide the miso-glazed salmon evenly between two plates and serve immediately.

Nutritional Values (per serving):

Calories: 280 | Fat: 11g | Saturated Fat: 2g | Cholesterol: 85mg | Sodium: 510mg | Carbohydrates: 7g | Fiber: 0g | Sugar: 4g | Protein: 37g

SHRIMP SCAMPI

Ingredients:

- 1 tbsp olive oil
- ½ lb shrimp, peeled and deveined
- 2 cloves garlic, minced
- ¼ cup dry white wine
- ¼ cup low-sodium chicken broth

- 1 tbsp lemon juice
- ¼ tsp red pepper flakes
- ¼ tsp salt
- ¼ tsp black pepper
- ¼ cup chopped fresh parsley

Instructions:

1. Using a large non-stick skillet, heat up the olive oil over a medium-high heat setting.
2. Place the shrimp into the pan and allow it to cook for approximately 2-3 minutes on each side until it turns pink in color and is fully cooked. Remove the shrimp from the frying pan and transfer them to a dish using a slotted spoon.
3. In the same skillet, add the garlic and cook it for about 1 minute or until it becomes fragrant.
4. In a saucepan, combine chicken broth, white wine, lemon juice, red pepper flakes, salt, and black pepper. Mix the ingredients thoroughly until the mixture starts to simmer.
5. Let the mixture cook for 3-4 minutes or until the sauce has reduced slightly to your desired consistency.
6. Once the sauce has reduced slightly, add the prawns back to the frying pan and continue cooking for another 1-2 minutes or until they are fully warmed through.
7. Stir in the chopped fresh parsley. Divide the shrimp scampi between two plates and serve.

Nutritional Values (per serving):

Calories: 210 | Fat: 9g | Saturated Fat: 1.5g | Cholesterol: 180mg | Sodium: 740mg | Carbohydrates: 3g | Fiber: 0g | Sugar: 1g | Protein: 29g

LEMON GARLIC BAKED TILAPIA

Ingredients:

- 2 (6 oz) tilapia fillets
- 1 tbsp olive oil
- 2 cloves garlic, minced
- ½ lemon, juiced
- ¼ tsp salt
- ¼ tsp black pepper
- ¼ tsp paprika
- ¼ cup chopped fresh parsley

Instructions:

1. Warm up the oven to a temperature of 400°F (200°C).
2. Cover a baking sheet with parchment paper, and then place the tilapia fillets on the baking sheet.
3. Combine minced garlic, lemon juice, olive oil, salt, black pepper, and paprika in a small bowl and mix all the ingredients together thoroughly. Blend well.
4. Spread the garlic sauce over the fillets of tilapia.
5. Cook the fish in the oven for a duration of 12 to 15 minutes or until it becomes tender enough to break apart effortlessly using a fork.
6. Garnish with chopped fresh parsley and serve.

Nutritional Values (per serving):

Calories: 230 | Fat: 10g | Saturated Fat: 1.5g | Cholesterol: 85mg | Sodium: 420mg | Carbohydrates: 3g | Fiber: 1g | Sugar: 0g | Protein: 34g

SHRIMP AND SPINACH STUFFED PORTOBELLO MUSHROOMS

Ingredients:

- 2 large Portobello mushroom caps, stems removed
- 1 tbsp olive oil
- ½ lb shrimp, peeled and deveined
- 2 cups baby spinach, chopped
- ¼ cup low-fat cream cheese
- ¼ cup grated Parmesan cheese
- ¼ tsp garlic powder
- ¼ tsp salt
- ¼ tsp black pepper

Instructions:

1. Warm up the oven to a temperature of 400°F (200°C). Put parchment paper on a baking sheet.
2. Place the Portobello mushroom caps on the prepared baking sheet, gill-side up.
3. Place a nonstick skillet on medium heat and warm up the olive oil until it's hot. Add the shrimp to the skillet and allow them to cook for approximately 2-3 minutes on each side until they are pink and cooked through. Ensure that the shrimp have turned a light pink color before removing them from the heat to indicate they are fully cooked. Remove the prawns from the pan and dice them into small pieces.
4. In the same skillet, add the chopped spinach and cook it for 1-2 minutes or until it wilts and becomes tender.
5. In a medium bowl, mix together the cooked shrimp, wilted spinach, cream cheese, Parmesan cheese, garlic powder, salt, and black pepper.
6. Spoon the shrimp and spinach mixture into the Portobello mushroom caps.
7. Bake the dish in the oven for 12-15 minutes or until the mushrooms are tender and the cheese has melted.
8. Divide the stuffed Portobello mushrooms evenly between two plates and serve immediately.

Nutritional Values (per serving):

Calories: 340 | Fat: 17g | Saturated Fat: 6g | Cholesterol: 180mg | Sodium: 800mg | Carbohydrates: 12g | Fiber: 2g | Sugar: 5g | Protein: 37g

TERIYAKI GLAZED SALMOND

Ingredients:

- 2 (6 oz) salmon fillets
- ¼ cup low-sodium soy sauce
- ¼ cup mirin
- ¼ cup honey
- ½ tsp grated ginger
- ½ tsp minced garlic

Instructions:

1. Before baking, it is recommended to warm up the oven to a

temperature of 400°F (200°C). Put parchment paper on a baking sheet.
2. Combine the soy sauce, mirin, honey, ginger, and garlic in a small saucepan. Heat the mixture over medium heat until it simmers, then continue cooking for 5 to 7 minutes until the sauce reaches a slightly thicker consistency.
3. Brush the teriyaki sauce on the salmon fillets and put them on the baking sheet.
4. Put the salmon into the oven and cook it for around 10-12 minutes or until it becomes flaky and separates easily when poked with a fork. Brush with additional teriyaki sauce halfway through the cooking time.
5. Take out the cooked salmon from the oven and use a brush to apply the teriyaki sauce that is left over.
6. Divide the salmon evenly between two plates and serve immediately.

Nutritional Values (per serving):

Calories: 390 | Fat: 11g | Saturated Fat: 2g | Cholesterol: 95mg | Sodium: 720mg | Carbohydrates: 33g | Fiber: 0g | Sugar: 30g | Protein: 35g

SEAFOOD-STUFFED BELL PEPPERS

Ingredients:

- 2 large bell peppers, halved lengthwise and seeded
- ½ lb mixed seafood (shrimp, crab, scallops), cooked and chopped
- ½ cup cooked brown rice
- ¼ cup chopped onion
- ¼ cup chopped tomato
- ¼ cup chopped fresh parsley
- ¼ cup low-fat feta cheese, crumbled
- ¼ tsp salt
- ¼ tsp black pepper

Instructions:

1. Set the oven to 375°F (190°C). Line a baking sheet with parchment paper.
2. Place the bell pepper halves on the prepared baking sheet, cut side up.
3. Mix the cooked seafood, brown rice, onion, tomato, parsley, feta cheese, salt, and black pepper in a medium bowl.
4. Spoon the seafood mixture into the bell pepper halves, pressing down gently to pack the mixture in.
5. Roast the stuffed bell peppers in the oven for around 25-30 minutes or until the peppers are tender and the filling is heated completely.
6. Divide the stuffed bell peppers evenly between two plates and serve immediately.

Nutritional Values (per serving):

Calories: 290 | Fat: 5g | Saturated Fat: 2g | Cholesterol: 150mg | Sodium: 640mg | Carbohydrates: 29g | Fiber: 5g | Sugar: 8g | Protein: 30g

LEMON GARLIC SHRIMP AND ASPARAGUS

Ingredients:

- ½ lb shrimp, peeled and deveined
- ½ lb asparagus, trimmed
- 2 tbsp olive oil
- 2 cloves garlic, minced
- ½ lemon, juiced
- ¼ tsp salt
- ¼ tsp black pepper

Instructions:

1. Using a generously-sized non-stick skillet, warm up some olive oil over medium heat. Proceed by introducing the minced garlic, ensuring to stir it constantly for a minute.
2. Next, gently add the shrimp to the skillet, making sure to cook it for 2 to 3 minutes on each side until it turns a delicate pink and has been cooked all the way through. After the shrimp is cooked, take it out of the skillet and keep it aside.
3. Now, you can introduce the asparagus to the same skillet, cooking it for 4 to 5 minutes so that it turns tender but still maintains some of its crispness. Once the asparagus is ready, add back the shrimp and stir in the lemon juice, salt, and black pepper.
4. Give everything a good mix, cooking it for another 1 to 2 minutes until all the flavors have melded together, and everything is evenly heated.
5. Divide the shrimp and asparagus evenly between two plates and serve immediately.

Nutritional Values (per serving):

Calories: 270 | Fat: 15g | Saturated Fat: 2g | Cholesterol: 180mg | Sodium: 590mg | Carbohydrates: 8g | Fiber: 3g | Sugar: 3g | Protein: 27g

---

PESTO BAKED SCALLOPS

Ingredients:

- ½ lb large scallops
- ¼ cup prepared basil pesto
- ¼ cup panko breadcrumbs
- ¼ cup grated Parmesan cheese
- 1 tbsp olive oil

Instructions:

1. To start, you should preheat your oven to 400°F (200°C). Following this, prepare your baking sheet by covering it with parchment paper.
2. Prepare the baking dish and arrange the scallops in a way that they are not overlapping, forming a single layer.
3. Spread a thin layer of basil pesto over each scallop using a spoon or brush.
4. Mix the panko breadcrumbs, Parmesan cheese, and olive oil in a small bowl. Sprinkle the breadcrumb mixture evenly over the scallops to create a crispy and flavorful crust.
5. Bake the scallops in the oven for 12-15 minutes or until they are cooked through and the breadcrumb topping is golden brown.

6. Divide the baked scallops evenly between two plates and serve immediately.

Nutritional Values (per serving):

Calories: 330 | Fat: 19g | Saturated Fat: 4g | Cholesterol: 55mg | Sodium: 700mg | Carbohydrates: 13g | Fiber: 1g | Sugar: 1g | Protein: 25g

TILAPIA WITH LEMON CAPER SAUCE

Ingredients:

- 2 (6 oz) tilapia fillets
- 1 tbsp olive oil
- ¼ cup low-sodium chicken broth
- ¼ cup lemon juice
- 2 tbsp capers, drained
- ¼ tsp salt
- ¼ tsp black pepper

Instructions:

1. Start by heating up some olive oil in a non-stick pan over medium-high heat. Place the tilapia fillets gently into the frying pan and cook them until they are crispy and golden brown on each side, which should take around 3 to 4 minutes. Be sure to cook the ingredients thoroughly until they are fully cooked to ensure they are safe to eat.
2. The tilapia should be put on a plate and covered with aluminum foil to keep it warm.
3. Add the chicken broth, lemon juice, capers, salt, and black pepper in the same skillet. Bring the mixture to a simmer and cook it for 2-3 minutes or until the sauce has reduced slightly to your desired consistency.
4. Spoon the lemon caper sauce over the cooked tilapia fillets.
5. Divide the tilapia fillets evenly between two plates and serve immediately.

Nutritional Values (per serving):

Calories: 230 | Fat: 10g | Saturated Fat: 1.5g | Cholesterol: 85mg | Sodium: 540mg | Carbohydrates: 3g | Fiber: 0g | Sugar: 1g | Protein: 34g

SPICY ORANGE GLAZED SHRIMP

Ingredients:

- ½ lb shrimp, peeled and deveined
- ¼ cup fresh orange juice
- 1 tbsp low-sodium soy sauce
- 1 tbsp honey
- ¼ tsp red pepper flakes
- 1 tbsp olive oil
- ¼ tsp salt
- ¼ tsp black pepper

Instructions:

1. Mix the soy sauce, orange juice, honey, and crushed red pepper in a small bowl. Keep it aside.
2. Heat up the olive oil in a non-stick skillet over medium-high heat.
3. To prepare the shrimp, add a pinch of salt and a sprinkle of black pepper, then cook each side for approximately 2-3 minutes until they turn a pink color and are fully cooked.

4. Add the orange sauce to the skillet containing shrimp, and cook for an additional 1-2 minutes until the sauce thickens a bit and completely covers the shrimp.
5. Divide the cooked shrimp evenly between two plates and serve immediately.

Nutritional Values (per serving):

Calories: 240 | Fat: 9g | Saturated Fat: 1.5g | Cholesterol: 180mg | Sodium: 660mg | Carbohydrates: 13g | Fiber: 0g | Sugar: 11g | Protein: 27g

POACHED COD WITH TOMATO SALSA

Ingredients:

- 2 (6 oz) cod fillets
- 1 cup low-sodium vegetable broth
- 1 cup chopped tomatoes
- ¼ cup chopped red onion
- ¼ cup chopped fresh cilantro
- 1 tbsp lime juice
- ¼ tsp salt
- ¼ tsp black pepper

Instructions:

1. Bring the vegetable broth to a simmer over medium heat in a medium saucepan. Carefully place the cod fillets into the saucepan, making sure that they are completely submerged in the broth. Simmer the fish for 5-7 minutes or until it flakes easily with a fork. Once done, remove the cod from the broth and set it aside on a separate plate.
2. Mix the chopped tomatoes, red onion, cilantro, lime juice, salt, and black pepper in a medium bowl to create the salsa.
3. Divide the poached cod fillets evenly between two plates, and top each fillet with a generous spoonful of tomato salsa.
4. Serve immediately.

Nutritional Values (per serving):

Calories: 170 | Fat: 1g | Saturated Fat: 0g | Cholesterol: 60mg | Sodium: 540mg | Carbohydrates: 9g | Fiber: 2g | Sugar: 5g | Protein: 30g

LOBSTER AND CORN CHOWDER

Ingredients:

- ½ lb cooked lobster meat, chopped
- 1 tbsp olive oil
- ¼ cup chopped onion
- ¼ cup chopped celery
- ¼ cup chopped red bell pepper
- ¼ cup all-purpose flour
- 2 cups low-sodium chicken broth
- 1 cup frozen corn kernels
- 1 cup of low-fat milk
- ¼ tsp salt
- ¼ tsp black pepper

Instructions:

1. Put a saucepan of significant size on medium heat and warm up the olive oil until it reaches a high temperature. Add the onion, celery, and red bell pepper to the skillet and cook for 4-5 minutes, stirring occasionally, until the vegetables are softened.

2. Add the flour to the vegetable mixture and cook for 1-2 minutes or until the flour turns light brown. Gradually pour in the chicken broth, then add the corn, milk, salt, and black pepper, whisking continuously.
3. Once the mixture has reached boiling point, it is advisable to lower the heat to a mild simmer. Stir the mixture occasionally during the cooking process, which should take around 10-12 minutes or until the chowder has reached the desired thickness.
4. Introduce the cooked lobster meat into the mixture and stir well, cooking for an additional 2-3 minutes until the lobster meat is thoroughly heated.
5. Divide the chowder evenly between two bowls and serve immediately.

Nutritional Values (per serving):

Calories: 420 | Fat: 12g | Saturated Fat: 2g | Cholesterol: 135mg | Sodium: 790mg | Carbohydrates: 47g | Fiber: 5g | Sugar: 12g | Protein: 34g

SOUPS RECIPES

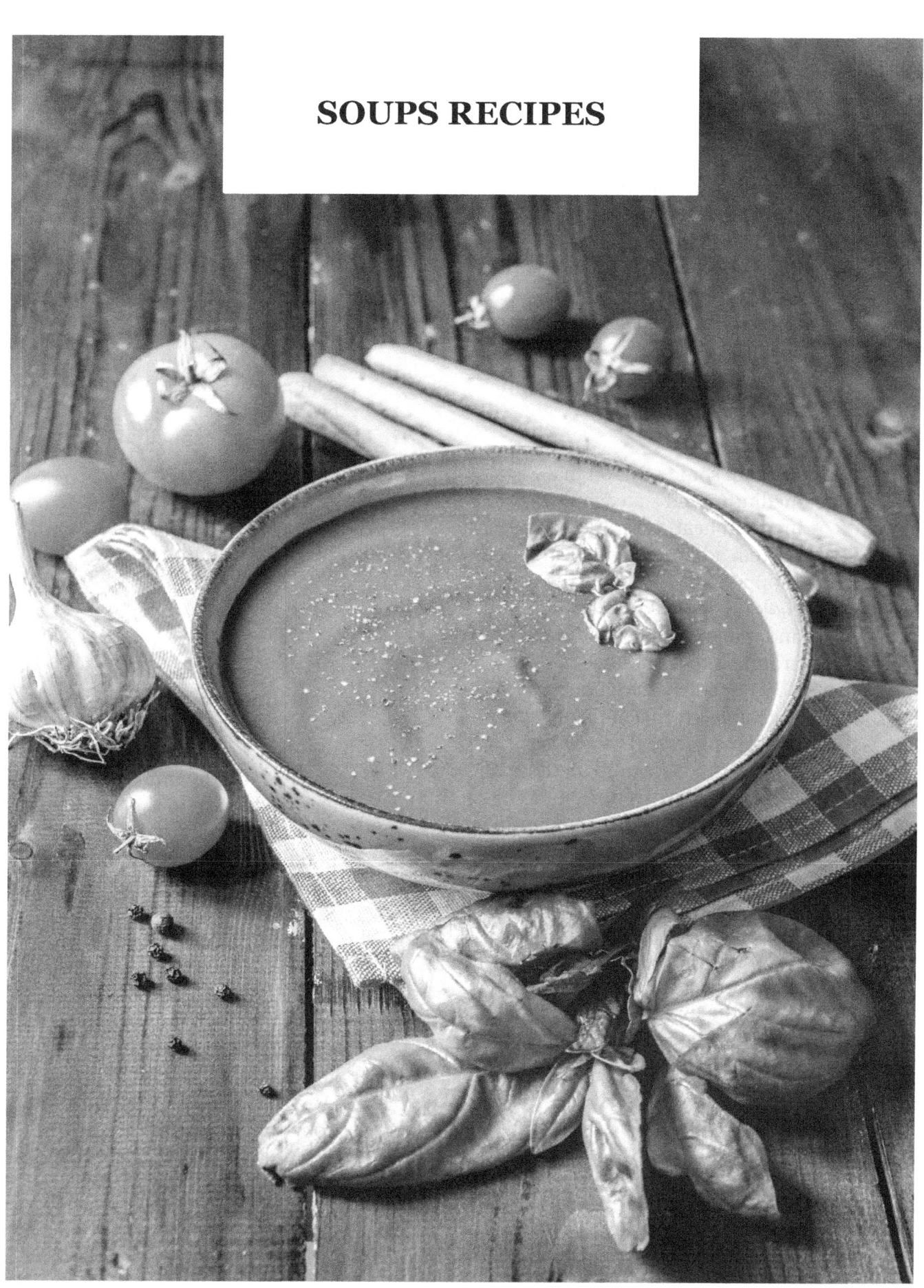

TOMATO BASIL SOUP

Ingredients:

- 1 tbsp olive oil
- ½ cup chopped onion
- 2 cloves garlic, minced
- 2 cups canned crushed tomatoes, no salt added
- 1 cup low-sodium vegetable broth
- ¼ cup chopped fresh basil
- ¼ tsp black pepper
- ¼ tsp salt

Instructions:

1. Heat up some olive oil in a medium-sized saucepan over medium heat. After the oil is heated, add the minced garlic and chopped onion to the pan, and cook them until they become soft and tender, which should take around 4 to 5 minutes.
2. Add the crushed tomatoes, vegetable broth, chopped basil, black pepper, and salt to the mixture and stir until all the ingredients are well combined.
3. The combination is heated until it reaches boiling point, then the heat is reduced, and the mixture is allowed to simmer for 30 minutes.
4. If you prefer a smoother soup, use an immersion blender to puree the mixture until it reaches your desired consistency.
5. After dividing the soup evenly into two bowls, it is now ready to be served.

Nutritional Values (per serving):

Calories: 160 | Fat: 7g | Saturated Fat: 1g | Cholesterol: 0mg | Sodium: 480mg | Carbohydrates: 23g | Fiber: 6g | Sugar: 13g | Protein: 5g

SPINACH AND WHITE BEAN SOUP

Ingredients:

- 1 tbsp olive oil
- ½ cup chopped onion
- 2 cloves garlic, minced
- 2 cups low-sodium vegetable broth
- 1 (15 oz) can cannellini beans, drained and rinsed
- ½ tsp dried thyme
- ¼ tsp salt
- ¼ tsp black pepper
- 2 cups packed fresh spinach

Instructions:

1. Heat up some olive oil in a medium-sized saucepan over medium heat. After the oil is heated, add the minced garlic and chopped onion to the pan, and cook them until they become soft and tender, which should take around 4 to 5 minutes.
2. Stir in the vegetable broth, cannellini beans, dried thyme, salt, and black pepper.
3. The mixture should be heated until it reaches boiling point, then cooled and simmered for ten minutes.
4. Add the spinach to the soup and cook for an additional 2-3 minutes or until the spinach has wilted. Stir the soup occasionally during this time.

5. After dividing the soup evenly into two bowls, it is now ready to be served.

Nutritional Values (per serving):

Calories: 240 | Fat: 7g | Saturated Fat: 1g | Cholesterol: 0mg | Sodium: 490mg | Carbohydrates: 36g | Fiber: 8g | Sugar: 4g | Protein: 12g

SPICED LENTIL SOUP

Ingredients:

- 1 tbsp olive oil
- ½ cup chopped onion
- ½ cup chopped carrots
- ½ cup chopped celery
- ½ cup dried green lentils, rinsed
- 2 cups low-sodium vegetable broth
- ½ tsp ground cumin
- ¼ tsp ground turmeric
- ¼ tsp paprika
- ¼ tsp salt
- ¼ tsp black pepper

Instructions:

1. Place a medium pot over medium heat and warm the olive oil until it's heated through. Add the chopped onion, carrots, and celery to the pot and cook for 4-5 minutes, stirring occasionally, until the vegetables have softened.
2. Stir in the lentils, vegetable broth, cumin, turmeric, paprika, salt, and black pepper.
3. Apply heat to the mixture until it comes to a boil, then decrease the temperature and let it simmer for around 25-30 minutes until the lentils are tender.
4. After dividing the soup evenly into two bowls, it is now ready to be served.

Nutritional Values (per serving):

Calories: 280 | Fat: 7g | Saturated Fat: 1g | Cholesterol: 0mg | Sodium: 480mg | Carbohydrates: 41g | Fiber: 16g | Sugar: 6g | Protein: 16g

MUSHROOM BARLEY SOUP

Ingredients:

- 1 tbsp olive oil
- ½ cup chopped onion
- ½ cup chopped celery
- ½ cup chopped carrots
- ½ lb fresh mushrooms, sliced
- ¼ cup pearl barley rinsed
- 3 cups low-sodium vegetable broth
- ¼ tsp dried thyme
- ¼ tsp salt
- ¼ tsp black pepper

Instructions:

1. Place a medium pot over medium heat and warm the olive oil until it's heated through. Add the chopped onion, celery, and carrots to a pot and cook for 4-5 minutes, stirring occasionally, until the vegetables have softened.
2. Add the sliced mushrooms to the pot and cook for an additional 3-4 minutes, stirring occasionally,

until the mushrooms have released their liquid and are slightly browned.
3. Stir in the barley, vegetable broth, thyme, salt, and black pepper.
4. The mixture should be brought to a boil before being reduced in heat and simmer for 40 to 45 minutes or until the barley is soft and tender.
5. After dividing the soup evenly into two bowls, it is now ready to be served.

Nutritional Values (per serving):

Calories: 250 | Fat: 7g | Saturated Fat: 1g | Cholesterol: 0mg | Sodium: 480mg | Carbohydrates: 42g | Fiber: 9g | Sugar: 7g | Protein: 9g

BUTTERNUT SQUASH AND APPLE SOUP

Ingredients:

- 1 tbsp olive oil
- ½ cup chopped onion
- ½ cup chopped celery
- ½ cup chopped carrots
- ½ lb butternut squash peeled and cubed
- 1 medium apple, peeled, cored, and chopped
- 2 cups low-sodium vegetable broth
- ¼ tsp ground cinnamon
- ¼ tsp ground nutmeg
- ¼ tsp salt
- ¼ tsp black pepper

Instructions:

1. Place a medium pot over medium heat and warm the olive oil until it's heated through. Add the chopped onion, carrots, and celery to the pot and cook for 4-5 minutes, stirring occasionally, until the vegetables have softened.
2. Add the butternut squash, apple, vegetable broth, cinnamon, nutmeg, salt, and black pepper to the pot and stir until all the ingredients are well combined.
3. Apply heat to the mixture until it comes to a boil, then decrease the temperature and let it simmer for around 20-25 minutes until the squash is tender.
4. Use an immersion blender to blend the soup until it reaches a smooth and creamy consistency.
5. After dividing the soup evenly into two bowls, it is now ready to be served.

Nutritional Values (per serving):

Calories: 210 | Fat: 7g | Saturated Fat: 1g | Cholesterol: 0mg | Sodium: 480mg | Carbohydrates: 38g | Fiber: 6g | Sugar: 15g | Protein: 3g

CHICKEN AND VEGETABLE SOUP

Ingredients:

- 1 tbsp olive oil
- ½ cup chopped onion
- ½ cup chopped carrots
- ½ cup chopped celery
- 2 cups low-sodium chicken broth
- ½ lb cooked chicken breast, diced
- ½ cup frozen peas

- ¼ tsp dried thyme
- ¼ tsp salt
- ¼ tsp black pepper

Instructions:

1. Place a medium pot over medium heat and warm the olive oil until it's heated through. Add the chopped onion, carrots, and celery to a pot and cook for 4-5 minutes, stirring occasionally, until the vegetables have softened.
2. Add the chicken broth, diced chicken, frozen peas, thyme, salt, and black pepper to the pot and stir until all the ingredients are well combined.
3. Apply heat to the mixture until it comes to a boil, then decrease the temperature and let it simmer for around 15 to 20 minutes or until the veggies are fork-tender.
4. Ladle the soup into two bowls, making sure to portion it evenly, and serve immediately.

Nutritional Values (per serving):

Calories: 290 | Fat: 9g | Saturated Fat: 2g | Cholesterol: 80mg | Sodium: 480mg | Carbohydrates: 18g | Fiber: 4g | Sugar: 5g | Protein: 33g

CREAMY CAULIFLOWER SOUP

Ingredients:

- 1 tbsp olive oil
- ½ cup chopped onion
- ½ cup chopped celery
- ½ cup chopped carrots
- ½ lb cauliflower, chopped
- 2 cups low-sodium vegetable broth
- ¼ cup unsweetened almond milk
- ¼ tsp salt
- ¼ tsp black pepper

Instructions:

1. Place a medium pot over medium heat and warm the olive oil until it's heated through. Add the chopped onion, celery, and carrots to a pot and cook for 4-5 minutes, stirring occasionally, until the vegetables have softened..
2. Stir in the cauliflower and vegetable broth. When the mixture reaches boiling point, turn the heat down, cover the pan, and let the mixture simmer for 15 to 20 minutes or until the cauliflower is soft.
3. Use an immersion blender to blend the soup until it reaches a smooth and creamy consistency.
4. Add the almond milk, salt, and black pepper to the pot and stir until all the ingredients are well combined.
5. After dividing the soup evenly into two bowls, it is now ready to be served.

Nutritional Values (per serving):

Calories: 160 | Fat: 7g | Saturated Fat: 1g | Cholesterol: 0mg | Sodium: 480mg | Carbohydrates: 22g | Fiber: 6g | Sugar: 8g | Protein: 6g

MINESTRONE SOUP

Ingredients:

- 1 tbsp olive oil
- ½ cup chopped onion
- ½ cup chopped celery
- ½ cup chopped carrots
- ½ cup chopped zucchini
- 2 cups low-sodium vegetable broth
- 1 (15 oz) can dice tomatoes, no salt added
- ½ cup canned kidney beans, drained and rinsed
- ½ cup small pasta (e.g., ditalini)
- ¼ tsp dried basil
- ¼ tsp dried oregano
- ¼ tsp salt
- ¼ tsp black pepper

Instructions:

1. Place a medium pot over medium heat and warm the olive oil until it's heated through.
2. Add the chopped onion, celery, carrots, and zucchini to a pot and cook for 4-5 minutes, stirring occasionally, until the vegetables have softened.
3. Stir in the vegetable broth, diced tomatoes, kidney beans, pasta, basil, oregano, salt, and black pepper.
4. Bring the mixture to a boil, then reduce the heat and let it simmer for around 10-15 minutes or until the pasta is cooked and the vegetables are tender. Stir the soup occasionally during this time.
5. After dividing the soup evenly into two bowls, it is now ready to be served.

Nutritional Values (per serving):

Calories: 320 | Fat: 7g | Saturated Fat: 1g | Cholesterol: 0mg | Sodium: 490mg | Carbohydrates: 55g | Fiber: 11g | Sugar: 9g | Protein: 14g

POTATO LEEK SOUP

Ingredients:

- 1 tbsp olive oil
- ½ cup chopped leeks (white and light green parts only)
- ½ cup chopped celery
- ½ cup chopped carrots
- ½ lb potatoes, peeled and cubed
- 2 cups low-sodium vegetable broth
- ¼ tsp dried thyme
- ¼ tsp salt
- ¼ tsp black pepper

Instructions:

1. Place a medium pot over medium heat and warm the olive oil until it's heated through. Add the chopped leeks, celery, and carrots to a pot and cook for 4-5 minutes, stirring occasionally, until the vegetables have softened.
2. Stir in the potatoes, vegetable broth, thyme, salt, and black pepper.
3. The mixture should be brought to a boil, then simmered for 20 to 25 minutes or until the potatoes are cooked.

4. Use an immersion blender to blend the soup until it reaches a smooth and creamy consistency.
5. After dividing the soup evenly into two bowls, it is now ready to be served.

Nutritional Values (per serving):

Calories: 220 | Fat: 7g | Saturated Fat: 1g | Cholesterol: 0mg | Sodium: 480mg | Carbohydrates: 37g | Fiber: 5g | Sugar: 5g | Protein: 5g

ROASTED RED PEPPER AND TOMATO SOUP

Ingredients:

- 1 tbsp olive oil
- ½ cup chopped onion
- ½ cup chopped celery
- ½ cup chopped carrots
- ½ lb roasted red peppers chopped
- 2 cups canned crushed tomatoes, no salt added
- 2 cups low-sodium vegetable broth
- ¼ tsp dried basil
- ¼ tsp salt
- ¼ tsp black pepper

Instructions:

1. Place a medium pot over medium heat and warm the olive oil until it's heated through. Add the chopped onion, celery, and carrots, and cook for 4-5 minutes, until softened.
2. Stir in the roasted red peppers, crushed tomatoes, vegetable broth, basil, salt, and black pepper.
3. Apply heat to the mixture until it comes to a boil, then decrease the temperature and let it simmer for around 15 to 20 minutes, or until the veggies are the desired tenderness and can be easily pierced with a fork.
4. Use an immersion blender to blend the soup until it reaches a smooth and creamy consistency.
5. After dividing the soup evenly into two bowls, it is now ready to be served.

Nutritional Values (per serving):

Calories: 190 | Fat: 7g | Saturated Fat: 1g | Cholesterol: 0mg | Sodium: 490mg | Carbohydrates: 30g | Fiber: 7g | Sugar: 13g | Protein: 5g

HEARTY VEGETABLE AND BARLEY SOUP

Ingredients:

- 1 tbsp olive oil
- ½ cup chopped onion
- ½ cup chopped carrots
- ½ cup chopped celery
- ½ cup chopped zucchini
- ½ cup chopped green beans
- ¼ cup pearl barley rinsed
- 3 cups low-sodium vegetable broth
- 1 (15 oz) can dice tomatoes, no salt added
- ¼ tsp dried thyme
- ¼ tsp salt
- ¼ tsp black pepper

Instructions:

1. Place a medium pot over medium heat and warm the olive oil until it's heated through. Add the chopped onion, carrots, celery, zucchini, and green beans to a pot and cook for 4-5 minutes, stirring occasionally, until the vegetables have softened.
2. Stir in the barley, vegetable broth, diced tomatoes, thyme, salt, and black pepper.
3. Apply heat to the mixture until it reaches boiling point, then lower the temperature and let it simmer for around 40 to 45 minutes or until the barley is soft and tender to the touch.
4. After dividing the soup evenly into two bowls, it is now ready to be served.

Nutritional Values (per serving):

Calories: 240 | Fat: 7g | Saturated Fat: 1g | Cholesterol: 0mg | Sodium: 490mg | Carbohydrates: 40g | Fiber: 9g | Sugar: 9g | Protein: 7g

WHITE BEAN AND KALE SOUP

Ingredients:

- 1 tbsp olive oil
- ½ cup chopped onion
- ½ cup chopped carrots
- ½ cup chopped celery
- 2 cups low-sodium vegetable broth
- 1 (15 oz) can cannellini beans, drained and rinsed
- ½ lb kale stemmed and chopped
- ¼ tsp dried rosemary
- ¼ tsp salt
- ¼ tsp black pepper

Instructions:

1. Place a medium pot over medium heat and warm the olive oil until it's heated through. Add the chopped onion, carrots, and celery to a pot and cook for 4-5 minutes, stirring occasionally, until the vegetables have softened.
2. Stir in the vegetable broth, cannellini beans, kale, rosemary, salt, and black pepper.
3. Apply heat to the mixture until it comes to a boil, then decrease the temperature and let it simmer for around 15-20 minutes until the kale is tender.
4. After dividing the soup evenly into two bowls, it is now ready to be served.

Nutritional Values (per serving):

Calories: 290 | Fat: 7g | Saturated Fat: 1g | Cholesterol: 0mg | Sodium: 480mg | Carbohydrates: 45g | Fiber: 11g | Sugar: 5g | Protein: 15g

CREAMY MUSHROOM SOUP

Ingredients:

- 1 tbsp olive oil
- ½ cup chopped onion
- ½ cup chopped celery
- ½ cup chopped carrots
- ½ lb mushrooms, sliced
- 2 cups low-sodium vegetable broth

- ½ cup milk (dairy or non-dairy)
- ¼ tsp dried thyme
- ¼ tsp salt
- ¼ tsp black pepper

Instructions:

1. Place a medium pot over medium heat and warm the olive oil until it's heated through. Add the chopped onion, celery, and carrots, and cook for 4-5 minutes, until softened.
2. Incorporate the mushrooms into the mixture and continue cooking for another 4-5 minutes until they start to brown and release their juice.
3. Stir in the vegetable broth, milk, thyme, salt, and black pepper.
4. Apply heat to the mixture until it comes to a boil, then decrease the temperature and let it simmer for around 15-20 minutes until the vegetables are tender.
5. After dividing the soup evenly into two bowls, it is now ready to be served.

Nutritional Values (per serving):

Calories: 190 | Fat: 9g | Saturated Fat: 2g | Cholesterol: 5mg | Sodium: 480mg | Carbohydrates: 22g | Fiber: 4g | Sugar: 9g | Protein: 7g

SPICED RED LENTIL SOUP

Ingredients:

- 1 tbsp olive oil
- ½ cup chopped onion
- ½ cup chopped carrots
- ½ cup chopped celery
- ½ cup red lentils, rinsed
- 2 cups low-sodium vegetable broth
- ¼ tsp ground cumin
- ¼ tsp ground turmeric
- ¼ tsp salt
- ¼ tsp black pepper

Instructions:

1. Place a medium pot over medium heat and warm the olive oil until it's heated through. Add the chopped onion, carrots, and celery to a pot and cook for 4-5 minutes, stirring occasionally, until the vegetables have softened.
2. Stir in the red lentils, vegetable broth, cumin, turmeric, salt, and black pepper.
3. Apply heat to the mixture until it comes to a boil, then decrease the temperature and let it simmer for around 20 to 25 minutes or until the lentils are soft.
4. After dividing the soup evenly into two bowls, it is now ready to be served.

Nutritional Values (per serving):

Calories: 260 | Fat: 7g | Saturated Fat: 1g | Cholesterol: 0mg | Sodium: 480mg | Carbohydrates: 37g | Fiber: 15g | Sugar: 4g | Protein: 14g

ZUCCHINI AND CORN CHOWDER

Ingredients:

- 1 tbsp olive oil
- ½ cup chopped onion
- ½ cup chopped zucchini
- ½ cup frozen corn
- 2 cups low-sodium vegetable broth
- ½ cup milk (dairy or non-dairy)
- ¼ tsp dried thyme
- ¼ tsp salt
- ¼ tsp black pepper

Instructions:

1. Place a medium pot over medium heat and warm the olive oil until it's heated through. Add the chopped onion to a pan and cook for 4-5 minutes over medium heat, stirring occasionally, until it has softened.
2. Add the zucchini and corn to the pot and cook for an additional 4-5 minutes, stirring occasionally, until the zucchini has softened.
3. Add the vegetable broth, milk, thyme, salt, and black pepper to the pot and stir until all the ingredients are well combined.
4. Apply heat to the mixture until it comes to a boil, then decrease the temperature and let it simmer for around 10 to 15 minutes to allow the flavors to meld.
5. After dividing the soup evenly into two bowls, it is now ready to be served.

Nutritional Values (per serving):

Calories: 190 | Fat: 9g | Saturated Fat: 2g | Cholesterol: 5mg | Sodium: 480mg | Carbohydrates: 25g | Fiber: 4g | Sugar: 9g | Protein: 6g

MISO VEGETABLE SOUP

Ingredients:

- 2 cups low-sodium vegetable broth
- ½ cup chopped onion
- ½ cup chopped carrots
- ½ cup chopped zucchini
- ½ cup sliced mushrooms
- ½ cup cubed tofu
- ¼ cup white miso paste
- 2 cups water
- ¼ cup chopped green onions
- ¼ cup chopped fresh cilantro

Instructions:

1. In a medium saucepan, bring the vegetable broth to a boil. Add the chopped onion, carrots, zucchini, mushrooms, and tofu to a pot and cook over medium heat for 10-15 minutes, stirring occasionally, until the vegetables are tender.
2. In a separate bowl, whisk together the miso paste and water until the mixture is smooth and well combined. Mix the miso mixture together and pour it into the pot.
3. After whisking the miso paste and water together, continue cooking the soup for an additional 5 minutes to allow the flavors to meld together. Stir occasionally to prevent any sticking or burning on the bottom of the pot.
4. Put some green onions and parsley on top of each bowl of soup, then serve.

Nutritional Values (per serving):

Calories: 190 | Fat: 5g | Saturated Fat: 1g | Cholesterol: 0mg | Sodium: 510mg | Carbohydrates: 24g | Fiber: 4g | Sugar: 6g | Protein: 12g

CABBAGE AND POTATO SOUP

Ingredients:

- 1 tbsp olive oil
- ½ cup chopped onion
- ½ cup chopped potatoes
- 2 cups shredded cabbage
- 2 cups low-sodium vegetable broth
- ¼ tsp caraway seeds
- ¼ tsp salt
- ¼ tsp black pepper

Instructions:

1. Place a medium pot over medium heat and warm the olive oil until it's heated through. Add the chopped onion and potatoes to a pot and cook for 4-5 minutes over medium heat, stirring occasionally, until the vegetables have softened.
2. Stir in the cabbage, vegetable broth, caraway seeds, salt, and black pepper.
3. Apply heat to the mixture until it comes to a boil, then decrease the temperature and let it simmer for around 15 to 20 minutes or until the cabbage is soft.
4. After dividing the soup evenly into two bowls, it is now ready to be served.

Nutritional Values (per serving):

Calories: 210 | Fat: 7g | Saturated Fat: 1g | Cholesterol: 0mg | Sodium: 480mg | Carbohydrates: 34g | Fiber: 7g | Sugar: 6g | Protein: 5g

PEA AND MINT SOUP

Ingredients:

- 2 cups frozen peas
- 2 cups low-sodium vegetable broth
- ¼ cup chopped fresh mint
- ¼ tsp salt
- ¼ tsp black pepper
- ¼ cup crème fraîche or sour cream (optional)

Instructions:

1. In a medium saucepan, bring the vegetable broth to a boil. Add the frozen peas to the pot and cook for an additional 4-5 minutes, stirring occasionally, until the peas are heated through and tender.
2. Stir in the fresh mint, salt, and black pepper to the pot and stir until all the ingredients are well combined.
3. Use an immersion blender to blend the soup until it reaches a smooth and creamy consistency.
4. Portion the soup into two bowls and add a dollop of crème fraîche or sour cream as a garnish, if desired, before serving.

Nutritional Values (per serving, without crème fraîche):

Calories: 130 | Fat: 1g | Saturated Fat: 0g | Cholesterol: 0mg | Sodium: 490mg | Carbohydrates: 22g | Fiber: 8g | Sugar: 8g | Protein: 8g

POTATO AND LEEK SOUP

Ingredients:

- 1 tbsp olive oil
- ½ cup chopped leeks, white and light green parts only
- ½ cup chopped potatoes
- 2 cups low-sodium vegetable broth
- ¼ tsp dried thyme
- ¼ tsp salt
- ¼ tsp black pepper

Instructions:

1. Place a medium pot over medium heat and warm the olive oil until it's heated through. Add the chopped leeks to the pot and cook for another 4 to 5 minutes, stirring occasionally, until the leeks are soft.
2. Mix in the potatoes, veggie broth, thyme, salt, and black pepper.
3. Apply heat to the mixture until it comes to a boil, then decrease the temperature and let it simmer for around 15 to 20 minutes or until the potatoes become tender.
4. After dividing the soup evenly into two bowls, it is now ready to be served.

Nutritional Values (per serving):

Calories: 190 | Fat: 7g | Saturated Fat: 1g | Cholesterol: 0mg | Sodium: 480mg | Carbohydrates: 28g | Fiber: 3g | Sugar: 4g | Protein: 3g

CARROT AND GINGER SOUP

Ingredients:

- 1 tbsp olive oil
- ½ cup chopped onion
- ½ cup chopped carrots
- ½ tsp minced fresh ginger
- 2 cups low-sodium vegetable broth
- ¼ tsp salt
- ¼ tsp black pepper

Instructions:

1. In a medium saucepan, heat the olive oil over medium heat. Add the chopped onion, carrots, and ginger to the pot and cook for 4-5 minutes, stirring occasionally, until the vegetables are softened.
2. Stir in the vegetable broth, salt, and black pepper to the pot.
3. Once the vegetables have softened, bring the mixture to a boil. Reduce the heat and let the soup simmer for 15-20 minutes, stirring occasionally, until the carrots are tender.
4. Use an immersion blender to puree the soup until it reaches a smooth consistency. Be careful when blending hot liquids and ensure the soup has cooled slightly before blending.
5. Divide the pureed soup evenly between two bowls and serve immediately. You can garnish

with fresh herbs or a drizzle of olive oil if desired.

Nutritional Values (per serving):

Calories: 130 | Fat: 7g | Saturated Fat: 1g | Cholesterol: 0mg | Sodium: 480mg | Carbohydrates: 15g | Fiber: 3g | Sugar: 6g | Protein: 2g

VEGETABLE RECIPES

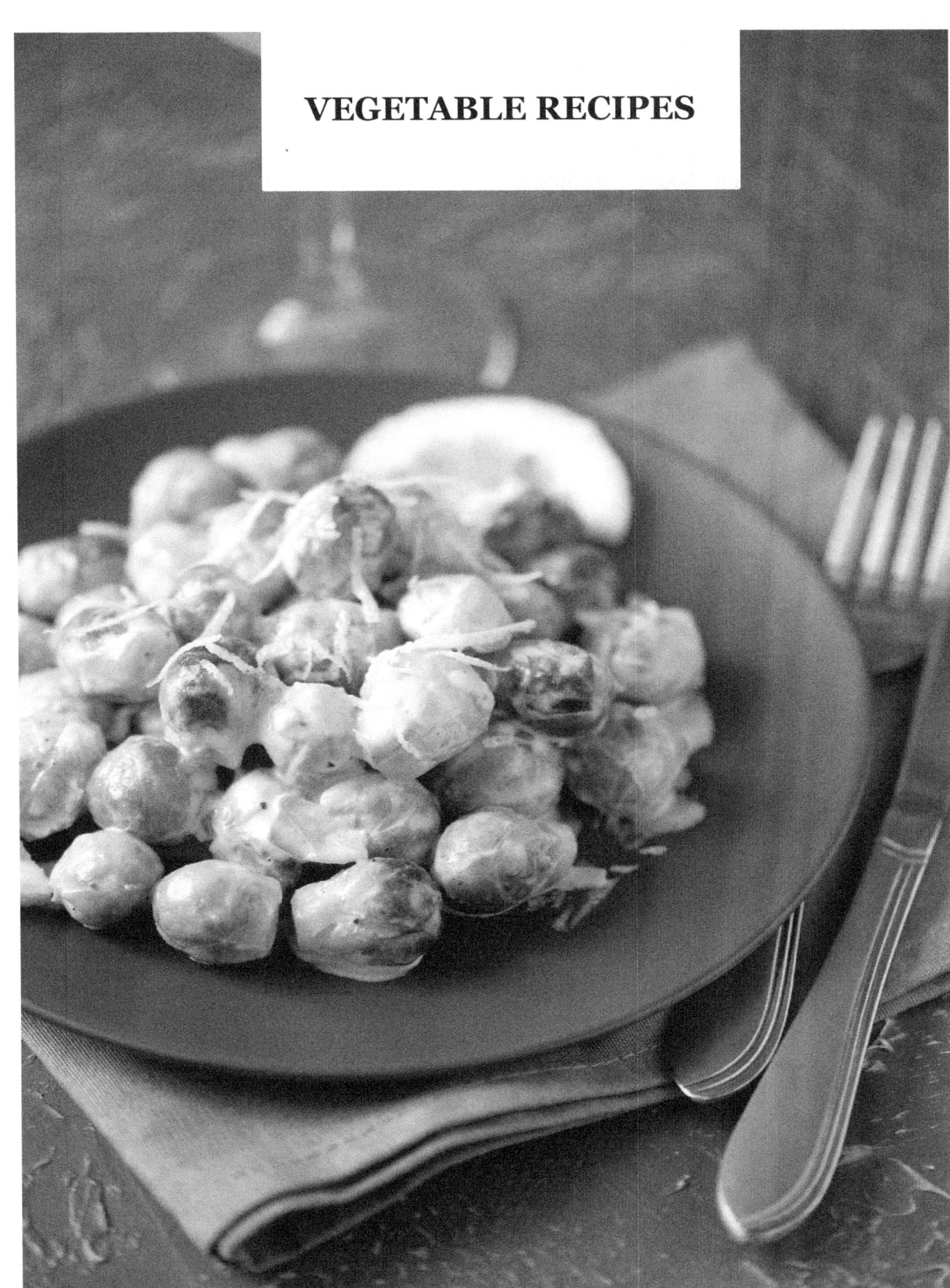

GARLIC-ROASTED BRUSSELS SPROUTS

Ingredients:

- 2 cups Brussels sprouts, halved
- 1 tbsp olive oil
- 2 cloves garlic, minced
- ¼ tsp salt
- ¼ tsp black pepper

Instructions:

1. Turn the oven's temperature up to 400 °F (200 °C). Line a baking sheet with parchment paper.
2. In a bowl, combine Brussels sprouts, olive oil, garlic, salt, and pepper. Toss to coat evenly.
3. Place the Brussels sprouts in one layer on the ready-to-use baking tray.
4. Place the vegetables on a baking sheet and roast them in the oven for 20-25 minutes, or until they are tender and slightly crispy. Serve immediately.

Nutritional Values (per serving):

Calories: 100 | Fat: 7g | Saturated Fat: 1g | Cholesterol: 0mg | Sodium: 330mg | Carbohydrates: 8g | Fiber: 3g | Sugar: 2g | Protein: 3g

CAULIFLOWER FRIED RICE

Ingredients:

- 1 tbsp olive oil
- ½ cup chopped onion
- ½ cup chopped bell pepper
- ½ cup chopped carrots
- 2 cups cauliflower rice
- ¼ cup low-sodium soy sauce
- ¼ tsp black pepper

Instructions:

1. Warm the olive oil in a sizable frying pan on medium heat. Include the onion, bell pepper, and carrots. Sauté for around 5-7 minutes until the vegetables become tender.
2. Add the cauliflower rice, soy sauce, and black pepper. Add the cauliflower to the pot and continue cooking for another 5-7 minutes, stirring occasionally, until the cauliflower becomes soft.
3. Ladle the cauliflower fried rice into two plates and serve immediately.

Nutritional Values (per serving):

Calories: 180 | Fat: 7g | Saturated Fat: 1g | Cholesterol: 0mg | Sodium: 480mg | Carbohydrates: 25g | Fiber: 6g | Sugar: 9g | Protein: 7g

BALSAMIC GLAZED CARROTS

Ingredients:

- 2 cups baby carrots
- 1 tbsp olive oil
- 2 tbsp balsamic vinegar
- ½ tsp dried thyme
- ¼ tsp salt
- ¼ tsp black pepper

Instructions:

1. Set the oven's temperature to 425°F (220°C). Line a baking sheet with parchment paper.
2. In a bowl, combine baby carrots, olive oil, balsamic vinegar, thyme, salt, and pepper. Toss to coat evenly.
3. Arrange the carrots in a single layer on the prepared baking sheet.
4. Roast the carrots in the preheated oven for 20-25 minutes, or until they are tender and caramelized. Serve immediately.

Nutritional Values (per serving):

Calories: 130 | Fat: 7g | Saturated Fat: 1g | Cholesterol: 0mg | Sodium: 420mg | Carbohydrates: 16g | Fiber: 4g | Sugar: 10g | Protein: 1g

CURRIED CHICKPEA AND SPINACH

Ingredients:

- 1 tbsp olive oil
- ½ cup chopped onion
- 1 clove garlic, minced
- ½ tsp curry powder
- ½ tsp ground cumin
- ¼ tsp salt
- ¼ tsp black pepper
- 1 cup canned chickpeas, drained and rinsed
- 2 cups baby spinach

Instructions:

1. Warm the olive oil in a sizable pan on medium heat. Incorporate the onion and sauté for 5 minutes until it becomes tender.
2. Stir in the garlic, curry powder, cumin, salt, and black pepper. Cook for 1-2 minutes, until fragrant.
3. Add the chickpeas and spinach. Cook the spinach for 3-4 minutes, stirring occasionally, until it is wilted.
4. Divide the curried chickpea and spinach mixture between two plates and serve.

Nutritional Values (per serving):

Calories: 210 | Fat: 9g | Saturated Fat: 1g | Cholesterol: 0mg | Sodium: 530mg | Carbohydrates: 27g | Fiber: 7g | Sugar: 6g | Protein: 8g

STUFFED BELL PEPPERS

Ingredients:

- 2 bell peppers, halved and seeds removed
- ½ cup cooked quinoa
- ½ cup black beans, drained and rinsed
- ¼ cup corn
- ¼ cup salsa
- ¼ tsp ground cumin
- ¼ tsp chili powder
- ¼ tsp salt
- ¼ cup shredded cheddar cheese

Instructions:

1. Set the oven's temperature to 375°F (190°C). Place the cut-side-up bell pepper halves on a baking sheet.

2. In a bowl, combine the quinoa, black beans, corn, salsa, cumin, chili powder, and salt.
3. Fill each bell pepper half with the quinoa mixture and top with shredded cheese.
4. Bake the peppers and cheese together for approximately 25 to 30 minutes or until the peppers have softened.
5. Serve right away.

Nutritional Values (per serving):

Calories: 220 | Fat: 6g | Saturated Fat: 2g | Cholesterol: 10mg | Sodium: 520mg | Carbohydrates: 33g | Fiber: 8g | Sugar: 6g | Protein: 10g

SWEET POTATO AND BLACK BEAN HASH

Ingredients:

- 1 tbsp olive oil
- 1 large sweet potato, diced
- ½ cup chopped onion
- ½ cup black beans, drained and rinsed
- ¼ tsp ground cumin
- ¼ tsp paprika
- ¼ tsp salt
- ¼ tsp black pepper
- 2 cups baby spinach

Instructions:

1. Warm the olive oil in a sizable frying pan on medium heat. Add the sweet potato and onion to the skillet and cook for 10-12 minutes, stirring occasionally, until the sweet potato is tender.
2. Stir in the black beans, cumin, paprika, salt, and black pepper to the skillet. Cook for an additional 3-4 minutes. Then, add the baby spinach to the skillet and cook for 2-3 minutes, stirring occasionally, until the spinach is wilted.
3. Divide the sweet potato and black bean hash between two plates and serve.

Nutritional Values (per serving):

Calories: 260 | Fat: 8g | Saturated Fat: 1g | Cholesterol: 0mg | Sodium: 490mg | Carbohydrates: 43g | Fiber: 11g | Sugar: 8g | Protein: 9g

LEMON-GARLIC GEREN BEANS

Ingredients:

- 2 cups green beans, trimmed
- 1 tbsp olive oil
- 2 cloves garlic, minced
- ¼ tsp salt
- ¼ tsp black pepper
- 1 tbsp lemon juice

Instructions:

1. Heat up a pot of water until it comes to a boiling point.
2. Blanch the green beans in boiling water for 3-4 minutes or until they reach a crisp-tender texture. Drain the beans and set them aside.
3. Add the olive oil to a skillet that has already heated to medium-high heat. Incorporate the garlic and cook for approximately 1-2

minutes or until it becomes fragrant.
4. Incorporate the green beans, salt, and black pepper into the dish and continue cooking for an additional 2-3 minutes or until the dish is thoroughly heated.
5. Stir in the lemon juice and serve immediately.

Nutritional Values (per serving):

Calories: 100 | Fat: 7g | Saturated Fat: 1g | Cholesterol: 0mg | Sodium: 300mg | Carbohydrates: 9g | Fiber: 3g | Sugar: 4g | Protein: 2g

SPICY ROASTED CAULIFLOWER

Ingredients:

- 2 cups cauliflower florets
- 1 tbsp olive oil
- ¼ tsp smoked paprika
- ¼ tsp cayenne pepper
- ¼ tsp salt
- ¼ tsp black pepper

Instructions:

1. Set the oven's temperature to 425°F (220°C). Prepare a baking sheet by lining it with parchment paper.
2. Combine the cauliflower florets, olive oil, smoked paprika, cayenne, salt, and black pepper in a bowl. Toss to coat evenly.
3. Arrange the cauliflower in a single layer on the prepared baking sheet.
4. Place the baking sheet with the cauliflower in the oven and roast for about 20-25 minutes until the florets become tender and develop a slightly charred appearance. Once done, serve immediately.

Nutritional Values (per serving):

Calories: 110 | Fat: 7g | Saturated Fat: 1g | Cholesterol: 0mg | Sodium: 330mg | Carbohydrates: 10g | Fiber: 4g | Sugar: 4g | Protein: 3g

STOVETOP RATATOUILLE

Ingredients:

- 1 tbsp olive oil
- ½ cup chopped onion
- ½ cup chopped bell pepper
- ½ cup chopped zucchini
- ½ cup chopped eggplant
- 1 cup canned diced tomatoes
- ¼ tsp dried basil
- ¼ tsp dried oregano
- ¼ tsp salt
- ¼ tsp black pepper

Instructions:

1. On medium heat, warm the olive oil in a large cooking pan. Add the onion, bell pepper, zucchini, and eggplant. Allow the vegetables to cook for approximately 7 to 8 minutes or until they have been softened.
2. Stir in the diced tomatoes, basil, oregano, salt, and black pepper. Bring the mixture to a simmer and continue cooking for an additional 15-20 minutes until the flavors have melded together

and the vegetables have become tender.
3. Divide the ratatouille between two plates and serve.

Nutritional Values (per serving):

Calories: 150 | Fat: 7g | Saturated Fat: 1g | Cholesterol: 0mg | Sodium: 470mg | Carbohydrates: 20g | Fiber: 6g | Sugar: 10g | Protein: 4g

PARMESAN ROASTED BROCCOLI

Ingredients:

- 2 cups broccoli florets
- 1 tbsp olive oil
- ¼ tsp salt
- ¼ tsp black pepper
- ¼ cup grated Parmesan cheese

Instructions:

1. Set the oven's temperature to 400°F (200°C). Line a baking sheet with parchment paper.
2. In a bowl, combine the broccoli florets, olive oil, salt, and black pepper. Toss to coat evenly.
3. Spread out the broccoli evenly in a single layer on the baking sheet that has been prepared.
4. Place the broccoli in the oven and roast for approximately 15-20 minutes or until it has become tender and slightly crispy.
5. Take the roasted broccoli out of the oven and sprinkle a generous amount of Parmesan cheese on top. Serve immediately.
6. Serve right away.

Nutritional Values (per serving):

Calories: 150 | Fat: 10g | Saturated Fat: 2g | Cholesterol: 5mg | Sodium: 480mg | Carbohydrates: 10g | Fiber: 4g | Sugar: 2g | Protein: 8g

GREEN BEANS ALMONDINE

Ingredients:

- 1 cup fresh green beans, trimmed
- 1 tbsp olive oil
- ¼ cup sliced almonds
- 1 small garlic clove, minced
- ¼ tsp salt
- ¼ tsp black pepper
- 1 tsp fresh lemon juice

Instructions:

1. Place the green beans in a steamer basket and steam them over boiling water for about 5 to 7 minutes or until they become tender-crisp. Once done, remove the steamer basket from the heat and set aside the green beans.
2. Olive oil should be heated in a sizable skillet over medium heat. Add the sliced almonds to the pan and cook for 2-3 minutes while stirring frequently until they become lightly toasted.
3. Incorporate the chopped garlic into the pan and continue cooking for another 30 seconds or until the garlic becomes fragrant.
4. Incorporate the steamed green beans, salt, and black pepper into the skillet with the toasted almonds. Stir everything together and cook for an additional two to

three minutes until the dish is thoroughly heated.
5. Remove the skillet from heat, drizzle with fresh lemon juice, and serve.

Nutritional Values (per serving):

Calories: 210 | Fat: 18g | Saturated Fat: 2g | Cholesterol: 0mg | Sodium: 300mg | Carbohydrates: 10g | Fiber: 4g | Sugar: 3g | Protein: 5g

GARLIC MASHED CAULIFLOWER

Ingredients:

- 2 cups cauliflower florets
- 1 tbsp unsalted butter
- 1 small garlic clove, minced
- ¼ tsp salt
- ¼ tsp black pepper
- 1 tbsp chopped chives (optional)

Instructions:

1. Steam the cauliflower florets in a steamer basket over boiling water for 8-10 minutes until tender.
2. Take a small saucepan and place it on a stove over medium-low heat. Add the butter to the saucepan and allow it to melt slowly. Put the minced garlic into the pan and cook for around 1-2 minutes or until it releases its aroma.
3. In a food processor, combine the steamed cauliflower, garlic-butter mixture, salt, and black pepper. Process until smooth and creamy.
4. Once the cauliflower is mashed to the desired consistency, transfer it to a serving bowl. If desired, garnish with chopped chives. Serve the dish immediately.

Nutritional Values (per serving):

Calories: 100 | Fat: 7g | Saturated Fat: 4g | Cholesterol: 15mg | Sodium: 320mg | Carbohydrates: 8g | Fiber: 3g | Sugar: 3g | Protein: 3g

SAUTÉED SPINACH WITH GARLIC

Ingredients:

- 1 tbsp olive oil
- 2 cups fresh spinach
- 1 small garlic clove, minced
- ¼ tsp salt
- ¼ tsp black pepper

Instructions:

1. On medium heat, warm the olive oil in a large cooking pan. Incorporate the chopped garlic into the pan and continue cooking for another 30 seconds or until the garlic becomes fragrant.
2. Add the spinach to the skillet and stir occasionally until it wilts. This should take about 2 to 3 minutes.
3. Season the dish with salt and black pepper according to taste. Serve immediately.

Nutritional Values (per serving):

Calories: 80 | Fat: 7g | Saturated Fat: 1g | Cholesterol: 0mg | Sodium: 330mg |

Carbohydrates: 3g | Fiber: 1g | Sugar: 0g | Protein: 2g

SWEET AND SOUR RED CABBAGE

Ingredients:

- 2 cups thinly sliced red cabbage
- ½ small red onion, thinly sliced
- ¼ cup apple cider vinegar
- 1 tbsp olive oil
- 1 tbsp honey
- ¼ tsp salt
- ¼ tsp black pepper

Instructions:

1. Place a large skillet on a stove over medium heat and add the olive oil to it. Warm up the olive oil until it is heated through. Incorporate the red onion into the heated olive oil in the skillet. Cook the onion for 2-3 minutes or until it has been softened.
2. Add the red cabbage to the skillet with the softened red onion. Cook for 5-7 minutes while stirring occasionally until the cabbage has become softened.
3. Take a small bowl and whisk the apple cider vinegar, honey, salt, and black pepper together until they are well-combined. Pour the mixture over the cabbage and cook for another 2 to 3 minutes, until everything is hot and mixed well.
4. Serve the sweet and sour red cabbage as a side dish.

Nutritional Values (per serving):

Calories: 110 | Fat: 7g | Saturated Fat: 1g | Cholesterol: 0mg | Sodium: 320mg | Carbohydrates: 13g | Fiber: 2g | Sugar: 10g | Protein: 1g

OVEN-ROASTED ROOT VEGETABLE

Ingredients:

- 1 medium carrot, peeled and chopped
- 1 medium parsnip, peeled and chopped
- 1 small beet, peeled and chopped
- 1 small turnip, peeled and chopped
- 2 tbsp olive oil
- ¼ tsp salt
- ¼ tsp black pepper
- ¼ tsp dried rosemary

Instructions:

1. Set the oven's temperature to 425°F (220°C). Line a baking sheet with parchment paper.
2. Take a large bowl and mix together the chopped carrot, parsnip, beet, and turnip. Lightly coat with olive oil, then season with salt, ground black pepper, and dried rosemary. Toss to coat the vegetables evenly.
3. Arrange the vegetables on the baking sheet that has been prepared, making sure to spread them out evenly and in a single layer. Roast for 25-30 minutes, occasionally stirring, until tender and golden brown.
4. Serve the oven-roasted root vegetables as a side dish.

Nutritional Values (per serving):

Calories: 200 | Fat: 14g | Saturated Fat: 2g | Cholesterol: 0mg | Sodium: 320mg | Carbohydrates

EGGPLANT PARMESAN STACKS

Ingredients:

- 1 medium eggplant, sliced into ½-inch rounds
- ½ cup whole wheat breadcrumbs
- ¼ cup grated Parmesan cheese
- ¼ tsp garlic powder
- ¼ tsp salt
- ¼ tsp black pepper
- 1 large egg, beaten
- ½ cup marinara sauce
- ½ cup shredded mozzarella cheese
- 1 tbsp chopped fresh basil

Instructions:

1. Set the oven's temperature to 375°F (190°C). Line a baking sheet with parchment paper.
2. In a small dish, mix the breadcrumbs, Parmesan cheese, garlic powder, salt, and pepper. Dip each eggplant slice into the beaten egg, and then coat it with the breadcrumb mixture until it is fully covered. Place the covered eggplant slices on the baking sheet that has already been set up.
3. Place the coated eggplant slices on a baking sheet and bake them for 15-20 minutes, flipping them over once during the cooking process, until they become golden brown and tender.
4. Remove the eggplant slices from the oven and add a spoonful of tomato sauce and some mozzarella cheese on top of each slice.
5. Place the eggplant slices with the tomato sauce and mozzarella cheese back in the oven and continue baking for another 5 minutes or until the cheese has fully melted and has become slightly bubbly.
6. Garnish the eggplant Parmesan stacks with chopped fresh basil and serve.

Nutritional Values (per serving):

Calories: 270 | Fat: 12g | Saturated Fat: 5g | Cholesterol: 75mg | Sodium: 840mg | Carbohydrates: 30g | Fiber: 7g | Sugar: 8g | Protein: 13g

CREAMY POLENTA WITH ROASTED VEGETABLES

Ingredients:

- 1 cup yellow cornmeal
- 4 cups vegetable broth
- ¼ cup grated Parmesan cheese
- ¼ cup heavy cream
- ¼ tsp salt
- ¼ tsp black pepper
- 2 cups assorted vegetables (e.g., zucchini, cherry tomatoes, bell peppers), chopped
- 2 tbsp olive oil
- ¼ tsp dried thyme
- ¼ tsp garlic powder

Instructions:

1. Set the oven's temperature to 425°F (220°C). Line a baking sheet with parchment paper.
2. Place a large saucepan on a stove and pour the vegetable broth into it. Heat the broth over high heat until it reaches the boiling point. Slowly pour the cornmeal into the boiling vegetable broth while continuously whisking to prevent the formation of lumps in the mixture. Reduce the heat to a moderate simmer and continue cooking for 20 to 25 minutes, stirring occasionally, until the polenta has thickened and become smooth.
3. Stir in the Parmesan cheese, heavy cream, salt, and black pepper. Keep the polenta warm while preparing the vegetables.
4. In a large bowl, mix the chopped veggies, olive oil, dried thyme, and garlic powder until everything is evenly coated.
5. Arrange the vegetables in a single layer on the prepared baking sheet to ensure even cooking.
6. Roast for 15-20 minutes, occasionally stirring, until tender and golden brown.
7. Plate the creamy polenta and top it with the roasted vegetables. Serve immediately.

Nutritional Values (per serving):

Calories: 410 | Fat: 22g | Saturated Fat: 8g | Cholesterol: 40mg | Sodium: 1010mg | Carbohydrates: 46g | Fiber: 6g | Sugar: 6g | Protein: 10g

STUFFED PORTOBELLO MUSHROOMS

Ingredients:

- 4 large portobello mushroom caps
- 2 tbsp olive oil
- ¼ tsp salt
- ¼ tsp black pepper
- ½ cup cooked quinoa
- ½ cup chopped spinach
- ¼ cup crumbled feta cheese
- ¼ cup chopped sun-dried tomatoes
- ¼ cup chopped fresh basil
- 1 tbsp balsamic vinegar

Instructions:

1. Set the oven's temperature to 375°F (190°C). Line a baking sheet with parchment paper.
2. Ensure that the portobello mushroom caps are clean and remove their gills and stems. Salt and pepper the mushroom caps on both sides and brush them with olive oil. Place the mushroom caps gill-side up on the prepared baking sheet.
3. In a medium bowl, combine the cooked quinoa, chopped spinach, feta cheese, sun-dried tomatoes, and chopped basil. Mix well.
4. Stuff each portobello mushroom cap with an equal amount of the quinoa mixture, pressing down gently to fill the cap completely.
5. Bake the mushrooms until the mushrooms are soft, and the sauce is hot, about 15 to 20 minutes.

6. Drizzle the stuffed portobello mushrooms with balsamic vinegar and serve.

Nutritional Values (per serving):

Calories: 240 | Fat: 15g | Saturated Fat: 4g | Cholesterol: 15mg | Sodium: 570mg | Carbohydrates: 20g | Fiber: 4g | Sugar: 5g | Protein: 8g

ZUCCHINI FRITTERS

Ingredients:

- 2 cups grated zucchini
- ½ cup all-purpose flour
- ½ cup grated Parmesan cheese
- 1 large egg, beaten
- ¼ cup chopped green onion
- ¼ tsp salt
- ¼ tsp black pepper
- ¼ cup vegetable oil

Instructions:

1. Take the chopped zucchini and place it in a clean dish towel. Squeeze and press the zucchini in the towel to remove as much excess moisture as possible.
2. Combine the zucchini, flour, Parmesan cheese, egg, green onion, salt, and black pepper in a large bowl and mix well. Mix well to form a thick batter.
3. Place a large skillet on the stove over medium heat and add the vegetable oil to it. Heat the oil until it is warmed up. Drop heaping tablespoons of the zucchini batter into the skillet, flattening each fritter slightly with the back of a spoon.
4. Add the zucchini fritters to the skillet and cook for 3-4 minutes per side, or until they become golden brown and crisp. Once the zucchini fritters have been cooked, place them on a plate that has been lined with paper towels. This will help to absorb any excess oil.
5. Plate the zucchini fritters and serve them with your preferred dipping sauce.

Nutritional Values (per serving):

Calories: 260 | Fat: 18g | Saturated Fat: 4g | Cholesterol: 55mg | Sodium: 480mg | Carbohydrates: 16g | Fiber: 1g | Sugar: 2g | Protein: 9g

CHICKPEA AND VEGETABLE CURRY

Ingredients:

- 1 tbsp vegetable oil
- 1 medium onion, chopped
- 2 cloves garlic, minced
- 1 tbsp curry powder
- ¼ tsp ground turmeric
- ¼ tsp ground cumin
- ¼ tsp ground coriander
- ¼ tsp cayenne pepper
- 1 (15 oz) can chickpeas, drained and rinsed
- 1 (14.5 oz) can diced tomatoes
- 1 cup chopped zucchini
- 1 cup chopped bell peppers
- ½ cup coconut milk
- ½ cup vegetable broth
- ¼ tsp salt
- ¼ tsp black pepper
- ¼ cup chopped fresh cilantro

Instructions:

1. Heat the vegetable oil in a large skillet over medium heat. Incorporate the onion and garlic into the heated skillet and cook for 2-3 minutes until they have become softened.
2. Add the curry powder, turmeric, cumin, coriander, and cayenne pepper to the skillet and stir everything together. Cook the spices for 1 minute or until they become fragrant.
3. Incorporate the chickpeas, diced tomatoes, zucchini, bell peppers, coconut milk, vegetable broth, salt, and black pepper into the skillet with the onion and garlic. Mix everything together and bring the mixture to a boil. Reduce the heat to low and let it simmer for approximately 20-25 minutes or until the vegetables have become tender and the flavors have melded together.
4. Stir in the chopped cilantro and serve the chickpea and vegetable curry over rice or with flatbread.

Nutritional Values (per serving):

Calories: 270 | Fat: 12g | Saturated Fat: 6g | Cholesterol: 0mg | Sodium: 790mg | Carbohydrates: 33g | Fiber: 8g | Sugar: 9g | Protein: 9g

DESSERT RECIPES

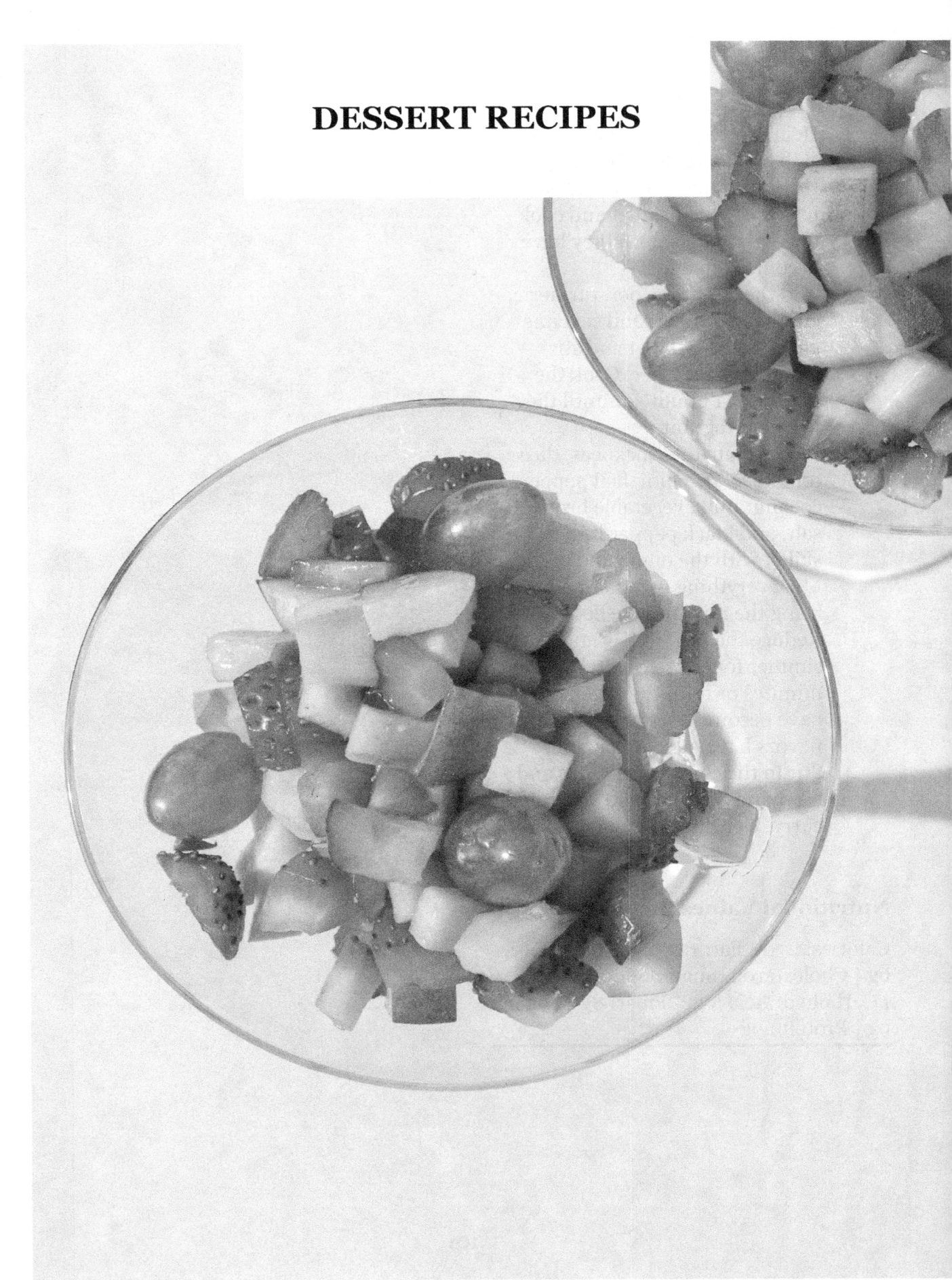

EASY FRUIT SALAD

Ingredients:

- 2 cups strawberries, hulled and halved
- 1 cup blueberries
- 1 cup raspberries
- 1 cup diced pineapple
- 1 cup diced kiwi
- 2 tbsp honey
- 1 tbsp fresh lime juice
- ¼ tsp lime zest

Instructions:

1. Put the strawberries, blueberries, raspberries, pineapple, and kiwi in a big bowl and mix them all together.
2. Take a small mixing bowl and combine the honey, lime juice, and lime zest. Whisk the ingredients together until they are thoroughly blended.
3. Once the fruit is prepared, pour the honey-lime dressing over it. Gently toss the fruit to ensure that it is evenly coated with the dressing.
4. Chill the fruit salad for at least 30 minutes before serving.

Nutritional Values (per serving):

Calories: 110 | Fat: 0.5g | Saturated Fat: 0g | Cholesterol: 0mg | Sodium: 5mg | Carbohydrates: 27g | Fiber: 4g | Sugar: 21g | Protein: 1g

CHOCOLATE AVOCADO MOUSSE

Ingredients:

- 2 ripe avocados
- ⅓ cup unsweetened cocoa powder
- ¼ cup honey
- ¼ cup unsweetened almond milk
- 1 tsp pure vanilla extract
- Pinch of salt
- Fresh berries, for serving

Instructions:

1. Put the avocado meat in a blender or food processor. Combine the cocoa powder, honey, almond milk, vanilla extract, and salt in a mixing bowl.
2. The ingredients should be smooth and creamy after blending, pausing occasionally to clean the sides of the blender as necessary.
3. Divide the chocolate avocado mousse among serving cups and chill for at least 1 hour.
4. Serve the mousse topped with fresh berries.

Nutritional Values (per serving):

Calories: 210 | Fat: 14g | Saturated Fat: 2g | Cholesterol: 0mg | Sodium: 50mg | Carbohydrates: 28g | Fiber: 7g | Sugar: 17g | Protein: 3g

BAKED CINNAMON APPLE SLICES

Ingredients:

- 4 medium apples, cored and sliced

- 2 tbsp unsalted butter, melted
- ¼ cup brown sugar
- ½ tsp ground cinnamon
- Pinch of salt

Instructions:

1. Set the oven's temperature to 375°F (190°C). Line a baking sheet with parchment paper.
2. Mix the melted butter, brown sugar, cinnamon, and salt with the apple slices in a big bowl.
3. Arrange the apple slices in a single layer on the prepared baking sheet.
4. Place the baking sheet with the apple slices in the oven and bake them for 20-25 minutes, or until they become tender and caramelized. Once done, remove the baking sheet from the oven and allow the apple slices to cool slightly before serving.

Nutritional Values (per serving):

Calories: 160 | Fat: 6g | Saturated Fat: 3.5g | Cholesterol: 15mg | Sodium: 35mg | Carbohydrates: 29g | Fiber: 4g | Sugar: 23g | Protein: 0g

COCONUT RICE PUDDING

Ingredients:

- ½ cup uncooked Arborio rice
- 1½ cups unsweetened coconut milk
- 1½ cups whole milk
- ¼ cup granulated sugar
- ¼ tsp salt
- ½ tsp pure vanilla extract
- ¼ tsp ground cinnamon
- ¼ cup unsweetened shredded coconut, toasted

Instructions:

1. In a medium saucepan, combine the Arborio rice, coconut milk, whole milk, granulated sugar, and salt. Place the mixture on a stove over medium heat and heat it until it begins to boil.
2. Lower the heat to a simmer and continue cooking the mixture, stirring occasionally, for approximately 35 to 40 minutes, until the rice is tender and the pudding has thickened.
3. After it has cooked, remove the pan from the heat source and blend in the vanilla extract and cinnamon powder, stirring until thoroughly combined.
4. Transfer the rice pudding to serving bowls and let cool for a few minutes. The pudding will become even thicker as it cools down.
5. Sprinkle the toasted shredded coconut over the rice pudding and serve warm or chilled.

Nutritional Values (per serving):

Calories: 280 | Fat: 13g | Saturated Fat: 10g | Cholesterol: 5mg | Sodium: 170mg | Carbohydrates: 36g | Fiber: 1g | Sugar: 19g | Protein: 5g

RASPBERRY LEMON SORBET

Ingredients:

- 3 cups fresh raspberries

- 1 cup granulated sugar
- 1 cup water
- ¼ cup fresh lemon juice
- 1 tsp lemon zest

Instructions:

1. Puree the raspberries in a mixer or food processor until they are smooth. Pass the puree through a fine mesh sieve to remove any seeds. Once the seeds have been removed, set the puree aside.
2. Combine the sugar and water in a small pot. Place the pot with the sugar and water mixture on a stove over medium heat. Stir the mixture occasionally and heat it until the sugar has fully dissolved. Once the sugar has dissolved completely, remove the pot from the heat and allow the syrup to cool down to room temperature.
3. Once the syrup has cooled down, add the raspberry puree, lemon juice, and lemon zest to it. Stir the mixture until everything is fully combined. Move the mixture to an ice cream maker and freeze it by following the maker's instructions.
4. Transfer the sorbet mixture to a jar with a tight-fitting lid. Place the jar in the freezer and allow the sorbet to freeze for at least 4 hours or until it becomes solid.

Nutritional Values (per serving):

Calories: 110 | Fat: 0g | Saturated Fat: 0g | Cholesterol: 0mg | Sodium: 0mg | Carbohydrates: 28g | Fiber: 2g | Sugar: 25g | Protein: 0g

CHOCOLATE-DIPPED BANANA BITES

Ingredients:

- 2 large bananas, peeled and sliced into ½-inch thick rounds
- 1 cup semisweet chocolate chips
- 1 tbsp coconut oil
- ¼ cup chopped nuts or shredded coconut, for garnish (optional)

Instructions:

1. Line a baking sheet with parchment paper. Arrange the banana slices in a single layer on the prepared baking sheet.
2. Take a microwave-safe bowl and combine the chocolate chips and coconut oil in it. Place the bowl with the chocolate chips and coconut oil in the microwave and heat it in 30-second intervals. Stir the mixture between each interval until the chocolate has melted and become smooth.
3. Using a fork, dip each banana slice into the melted chocolate until it is fully coated. Carefully shake off any excess chocolate and place the dipped banana slice back on the parchment paper.
4. If desired, sprinkle the chocolate-dipped banana slices with chopped nuts or shredded coconut before the chocolate sets.
5. Place the baking sheet with the chocolate-coated banana slices in the freezer for at least 30 minutes or until the chocolate has become firm. Once done, transfer the banana bites to an airtight

container and store them in the freezer.

Nutritional Values (per serving):

Calories: 130 | Fat: 7g | Saturated Fat: 4g | Cholesterol: 0mg | Sodium: 0mg | Carbohydrates: 18g | Fiber: 2g | Sugar: 12g | Protein: 1g

MINI FRUIT TARTS

Ingredients:

- 1 cup almond flour
- ¼ cup coconut oil melted
- 2 tbsp maple syrup
- 1 cup Greek yogurt
- ¼ cup honey
- 1 tsp pure vanilla extract
- 1 cup mixed fresh fruit (such as berries, kiwi, or diced peaches)

Instructions:

1. Set the oven's temperature to 350°F (175°C). Grease a 12-cup mini muffin pan.
2. In a medium-sized bowl, combine the almond flour, melted coconut oil, and maple syrup. Mix the ingredients together until a crumbly dough forms.
3. Press the crumbly dough into the bottom and up the sides of each muffin cup with your fingers until it forms a crust.
4. Place the muffin tin in the oven and bake the crusts for 10-12 minutes or until they become golden brown. Once the crusts have finished baking, remove the muffin tin from the oven and allow the crusts to cool completely in the pan.
5. In a small bowl, whisk together the Greek yogurt, honey, vanilla extract, and cinnamon until they are fully combined.
6. Once the crusts are cooled, carefully remove them from the pan. Place a spoonful of the yogurt mixture into each crust and add a layer of fresh fruit on top.
7. You can either serve the mini fruit tarts immediately or store them in the refrigerator until you are ready to serve them.

Nutritional Values (per serving):

Calories: 150 | Fat: 10g | Saturated Fat: 4g | Cholesterol: 0mg | Sodium: 15mg | Carbohydrates: 14g | Fiber: 1g | Sugar: 11g | Protein: 3g

LEMON BLUEBERRY CHIA PUDDING

Ingredients:

- ¼ cup chia seeds
- 1 cup unsweetened almond milk
- ¼ cup fresh lemon juice
- 2 tbsp honey
- ½ tsp lemon zest
- 1 cup fresh blueberries

Instructions:

1. Combine the chia seeds, almond milk, lemon juice, honey, and lemon zest in a medium bowl. Whisk thoroughly until well blended.
2. Cover the bowl with a lid and put it in the fridge for at least 4 hours, or until the chia seeds have

soaked up the liquid and the mixture has thickened.
3. Stir the chia pudding well and divide it among serving cups. Top with fresh blueberries and serve.

Nutritional Values (per serving):

Calories: 180 | Fat: 7g | Saturated Fat: 1g | Cholesterol: 0mg | Sodium: 65mg | Carbohydrates: 27g | Fiber: 7g | Sugar: 17g | Protein: 4g

STRAWBERRY BANANA SMOOTHIE BOWL

Ingredients:

- 1 cup frozen strawberries
- 1 medium banana, sliced and frozen
- ½ cup unsweetened almond milk
- ¼ cup Greek yogurt
- 1 tbsp honey
- Toppings: fresh fruit, granola, nuts, or seeds

Instructions:

1. Add frozen banana, almond milk, Greek yogurt, and honey to a blender or food processor. Blend the ingredients until they are smooth and creamy in consistency.
2. Once the smoothie has been blended to a creamy texture, transfer it to a bowl and arrange your preferred toppings over the surface. You can enjoy the smoothie immediately.

Nutritional Values (per serving):

Calories: 260 | Fat: 3g | Saturated Fat: 0g | Cholesterol: 5mg | Sodium: 115mg | Carbohydrates: 53g | Fiber: 6g | Sugar: 37g | Protein: 9g

MANGO COCONUT POPSICLES

Ingredients:

- 2 cups diced mango
- 1 cup unsweetened coconut milk
- ¼ cup honey
- ½ tsp pure vanilla extract
- Pinch of salt

Instructions:

1. In a mixer or food processor, mix the diced mango, coconut milk, honey, vanilla extract, and salt.
2. Blend until smooth and creamy.
3. Pour the mango mixture into the popsicle molds, making sure to leave a little room at the top for the mixture to grow.
4. Insert the sticks into the molds and then place the molds in the freezer for a minimum of 4 hours, or until the popsicles are thoroughly frozen.
5. Hold the molds of the frozen popsicles under warm running water for a few seconds to loosen them and remove the popsicles from the molds.

Nutritional Values (per serving):

Calories: 120 | Fat: 5g | Saturated Fat: 4g | Cholesterol: 0mg | Sodium: 40mg | Carbohydrates: 19g | Fiber: 1g | Sugar: 17g | Protein: 1g

PINEAPPLE COCONUT MACAROONS

Ingredients:

- 2 cups unsweetened shredded coconut
- ½ cup finely diced pineapple
- ⅓ cup granulated sugar
- ¼ cup all-purpose flour
- 2 large egg whites
- ½ tsp pure vanilla extract

Instructions:

1. Set the oven's temperature to 325°F (163°C). Line a baking sheet with parchment paper.
2. In a medium bowl, combine the shredded coconut, diced pineapple, granulated sugar, and flour. Mix the egg whites and vanilla extract into the mixture and stir until well combined.
3. Scoop tablespoon-sized mounds of the coconut mixture onto the prepared baking sheet. Using your fingers, gently press the mounds together until they stick together.
4. Place the macaroons in the oven and bake for approximately 20 to 25 minutes, or until they turn a golden brown color.
5. Let the macaroons cool for 5 minutes on the baking sheet before putting them on a wire rack to cool fully.

Nutritional Values (per serving):

Calories: 90 | Fat: 5g | Saturated Fat: 4g | Cholesterol: 0mg | Sodium: 15mg | Carbohydrates: 11g | Fiber: 1g | Sugar: 9g | Protein: 1g

ALMOND APRICOT BITES

Ingredients:

- 1 cup dried apricots
- 1 cup almonds
- ¼ cup unsweetened shredded coconut
- 1 tbsp honey
- ¼ tsp ground cinnamon
- Pinch of salt

Instructions:

1. In a food processor, combine the dried apricots, almonds, shredded coconut, honey, cinnamon, and salt. Process until the mixture is finely chopped and sticks together when pressed.
2. Shape the dough into 1-inch balls and place them onto a baking sheet that has been lined with parchment paper.
3. After shaping the almond apricot mixture into bites, refrigerate them for at least 30 minutes or until they become firm. For storage, place them in an airtight jar in the fridge to prevent exposure to air.

Nutritional Values (per serving):

Calories: 100 | Fat: 6g | Saturated Fat: 1g | Cholesterol: 0mg | Sodium: 10mg | Carbohydrates: 11g | Fiber: 2g | Sugar: 8g | Protein: 2g

BAKED CINNAMON APPLES

Ingredients:

- 4 large apples, cored and sliced
- ¼ cup packed brown sugar
- ¼ cup old-fashioned oats
- ¼ cup all-purpose flour
- ½ tsp ground cinnamon
- ¼ tsp ground nutmeg
- ¼ cup unsalted butter softened

Instructions:

1. Set the oven's temperature to 350°F (175°C). Grease a 9x13-inch baking dish.
2. Set the apple slices in the baking dish you just made.
3. Combine brown sugar, oats, flour, cinnamon, and nutmeg in a medium-sized bowl. Use a fork or your fingertips to incorporate the melted butter until the mixture reaches a coarse crumb-like texture.
4. Sprinkle the crumb topping over the apples.
5. Once the mixture has been transferred to a baking dish, place it in the oven and bake for approximately 45 to 50 minutes, or until the apples are tender and the top has turned a golden brown.
6. Serve warm.

Nutritional Values (per serving):

Calories: 210 | Fat: 8g | Saturated Fat: 5g | Cholesterol: 20mg | Sodium: 0mg | Carbohydrates: 34g | Fiber: 4g | Sugar: 23g | Protein: 1g

FRUIT KABOBS WITH HONEY YOGURT DIP

Ingredients:

- 2 cups mixed fruit (such as strawberries, pineapple, kiwi, and grapes)
- 1 cup Greek yogurt
- 2 tbsp honey
- ¼ tsp pure vanilla extract
- ¼ tsp ground cinnamon

Instructions:

1. Thread the mixed fruit onto wooden skewers and arrange it on a platter.
2. In a small bowl, whisk together the Greek yogurt, honey, vanilla extract, and cinnamon until they are thoroughly combined. Serve the fruit kabobs with the honey yogurt dip on the side.

Nutritional Values (per serving):

Calories: 100 | Fat: 0g | Saturated Fat: 0g | Cholesterol: 0mg | Sodium: 20mg | Carbohydrates: 22g | Fiber: 2g | Sugar: 18g | Protein: 4g

DARK CHOCOLATE BARK WITH DRIED FRUIT AND NUTS

Ingredients:

- 8 oz dark chocolate, chopped
- ½ cup mixed dried fruit (such as cranberries, raisins, and chopped apricots)

- ½ cup mixed nuts (such as almonds, pistachios, and walnuts), chopped
- Pinch of sea salt

Instructions:

1. Line a baking sheet with parchment paper.
2. In a bowl that can go in the microwave, heat the dark chocolate in 30-second bursts, stirring after each one, until it is smooth and melted.
3. Pour the melted chocolate onto the baking sheet that has been prepped and spread it out in a thin, even layer.
4. Sprinkle the mixed dried fruit and chopped nuts evenly over the chocolate. Using your fingers, lightly press the ingredients into the chocolate until they are partially submerged.
5. Once the toppings have been added, refrigerate the chocolate bark for at least 30 minutes or until it has become firm and set. After it has been set, break the chocolate bark into smaller pieces and store them in an airtight container in the refrigerator for future consumption.

Nutritional Values (per serving):

Calories: 160 | Fat: 10g | Saturated Fat: 4g | Cholesterol: 0mg | Sodium: 25mg | Carbohydrates: 18g | Fiber: 2g | Sugar: 12g | Protein: 2g

To receive your FREE eBook "The Anti-Inflammatory Cookbook" Scan this QR Code

COVERSION TABLES

Below are some basic conversion tables for the various units of measurement used in the recipes above. These conversions can be helpful when following a recipe or when scaling it up or down.

VOLUME CONVERSION

1 teaspoon (tsp)	5 milliliters (ml)
1 teaspoon (tsp)	15 milliliters (ml)
1 teaspoon (tsp)	30 milliliters (ml)
1 cup	240 milliliters (ml)
1 pint (pt)	473 milliliters (ml)
1 quart (qt)	946 milliliters (ml)
1 gallon (gal)	3.785 liters (l)

WEIGHT CONVERSION

1 ounce (oz)	28.35 grams (g)
1 pound (lb)	453.59 grams (g)

LENGTH COVERSION

1 inch (in)	2.54 centimeters (cm)
1 foot (ft) = 12 inches (in)	30.48 centimeters (cm)

TEMPERATURE CONVERSION

Fahrenheit (°F) to Celsius (°C): (°F - 32) x 5/9 = °C
Celsius (°C) to Fahrenheit (°F): (°C x 9/5) + 32 = °F

Example Conversions:
350°F = (350 - 32) × 5/9 = 176.67°C ≈ 175°C
425°F = (425 - 32) × 5/9 = 218.33°C ≈ 220°C

30 DAY MEAL PLAN

This 30-day meal plan provides you with a variety of breakfast, lunch, and dinner options, as well as snacks and desserts. Including a diverse selection of recipes in your diet can provide you with a variety of flavors and nutrients, promoting a well-rounded and delicious eating experience. It is important to keep in mind that adjusting portion sizes and ingredients to meet your individual dietary needs and preferences is crucial for maintaining a healthy and balanced diet. Combining all the recipes in this cookbook can make a 1900-day meal plan.

Day 1

Breakfast: Banana Oat Pancakes

Snack: Spicy Roasted Chickpeas

Lunch: Turkey Meatballs with Garlic-Roasted Brussels Sprouts

Snack: Apple Slices with Almond Butter

Dinner: Lemon Garlic Baked Cod with Green Beans Almondine

Dessert: Easy Fruit Salad

Day 2

Breakfast: Spinach and Mushroom Egg White Scramble

Snack: Greek Yogurt Ranch Dip with Veggies

Lunch: Pork Tenderloin with Balsamic Glaze and Cauliflower Fried Rice

Snack: Mini Caprese Skewers

Dinner: Spiced Lentil Soup with a Veggie and Hummus Wrap

Dessert: Chocolate Avocado Mousse

Day 3

Breakfast: Overnight Chia Pudding

Snack: Celery Sticks with Cream Cheese and Everything Bagel Seasoning

Lunch: Beef Stir-Fry with Broccoli and Balsamic Glazed Carrots

Snack: Avocado-Stuffed Cherry Tomatoes

Dinner: Shrimp and Veggie Stir-Fry with Curried Chickpea and Spinach

Dessert: Baked Cinnamon Apple Slices

Day 4

Breakfast: Avocado and Tomato Toast

Snack: Cucumber Slices with Hummus

Lunch: Baked Chicken Fajita Stuffed Peppers with Sweet Potato and Black Bean Hash

Snack: Ants on a Log

Dinner: Spinach and White Bean Soup with Lemon-Garlic Green Beans

Dessert: Coconut Rice Pudding

Day 5

Breakfast: Apple Cinnamon Quinoa Breakfast Bowl

Snack: Easy Edamame

Lunch: Greek-Style Grilled Chicken with Garlic Mashed Cauliflower

Snack: Peanut Butter and Chocolate Rice Cakes

Dinner: Pan-Seared Scallops with Garlic Spinach and Sautéed Spinach with Garlic

Dessert: Raspberry Lemon Sorbet

Day 6

Breakfast: Veggie and Egg Breakfast Burrito

Snack: Spinach and Artichoke Dip

Lunch: Balsamic-Glazed Pork Chops with Stovetop Ratatouille

Snack: Fruit Kabobs with Honey-Yogurt Drip

Dinner: Salmon with Dill Yogurt Sauce and Parmesan Roasted Broccoli

Dessert: Chocolate-Dipped Banana Bites

Day 7

Breakfast: Greek Yogurt and Berry Parfait

Snack: Sliced Turkey and Cheese Roll-Ups

Lunch: Beef and Vegetable Stir-Fry with Spicy Roasted Cauliflower

Snack: Popcorn with Nutritional Yeast

Dinner: Crab Cakes with Lemon Aioli and Oven-Roasted Root Vegetables

Dessert: Mini Fruit Tarts

Day 8

Breakfast: Peanut Butter and Banana Smoothie

Snack: Bell Pepper Nachos

Lunch: Slow Cooker Beef Stew with Green Beans Almondine

Snack: Veggie Pinwheels

Dinner: One-Pan Shrimp and Asparagus with Sweet and Sour Red Cabbage

Dessert: Lemon Blueberry Chia Pudding

Day 9

Breakfast: Vegetable Omelet

Snack: Frozen Yogurt Bark

Lunch: Sheet Pan Sausage and Vegetables with Garlic-Roasted Brussels Sprouts

Snack: Chocolate Banana Bites

Dinner: Baked Tilapia with Mediterranean Salsa and Sautéed Spinach with Garlic

Dessert: Strawberry Banana Smoothie Bowl

Day 10

Breakfast: Berry Oatmeal

Snack: Smoked Salmon and Cream Cheese Cucumber Bites

Lunch: Chicken and Rice Stuffed Bell Peppers with Curried Chickpea and Spinach

Snack: Cheese and Crackers

Dinner: Easy Clam Spaghetti with Stovetop Ratatouille

Dessert: Mango Coconut Popsicles

Day 11

Breakfast: Tropical Green Smoothie

Snack: Spicy Roasted Chickpeas

Lunch: Spaghetti Squash Bolognese with Balsamic Glazed Carrots

Snack: Apple Slices with Almond Butter

Dinner: Seared Ahi Tuna with Mango Salsa and Lemon-Garlic Green Beans

Dessert: Pineapple Coconut Macaroons

Day 12

Breakfast: Cottage Cheese and Fruit Bowl

Snack: Greek Yogurt Ranch Dip with Veggies

Lunch: Garlic Herb Pork Tenderloin with Cauliflower Fried Rice

Snack: Mini Caprese Skewers

Dinner: Seafood Paella with Garlic Mashed Cauliflower

Dessert: Almond Apricot Bites

Day 13

Breakfast: Multigrain Waffles with Fruit

Snack: Celery Sticks with Cream Cheese and Everything Bagel Seasoning

Lunch: Chicken and Broccoli Stir-Fry with Sweet Potato and Black Bean Hash

Snack: Avocado-Stuffed Cherry Tomatoes

Dinner: Baked Cod with Cherry Tomatoes and Olives with Parmesan Roasted Broccoli

Dessert: Baked Cinnamon Apples

Day 14

Breakfast: Almond Butter and Apple Rice Cakes

Snack: Cucumber Slices with Hummus

Lunch: Turkey Meatball Subs with Spicy Roasted Cauliflower

Snack: Ants on a Log

Dinner: Garlic Butter Scallops with Oven-Roasted Root Vegetables

Dessert: Fruit Kabobs with Honey Yogurt Dip

Day 15

Breakfast: Spinach, Tomato, and Mozzarella Frittata

Snack: Easy Edamame

Lunch: Grilled Portobello Mushroom Burgers with Stovetop Ratatouille

Snack: Peanut Butter and Chocolate Rice Cakes

Dinner: Lemon Herb Baked Salmon with Sautéed Spinach with Garlic

Dessert: Dark Chocolate Bark with Dried Fruit and Nuts

Day 16

Breakfast: Smoked Salmon and Avocado Rice Cake

Snack: Spinach and Artichoke Dip

Lunch: Greek Chicken Pita Pockets with Garlic-Roasted Brussels Sprouts

Snack: Fruit Kabobs with Honey-Yogurt Drip

Dinner: Spicy Cajun Shrimp Skillet with Green Beans Almondine

Dessert: Easy Fruit Salad

Day 17

Breakfast: Turkey Sausage and Veggie Scramble

Snack: Sliced Turkey and Cheese Roll-Ups

Lunch: Philly Cheesesteak Stuffed Peppers with Cauliflower Fried Rice

Snack: Popcorn with Nutritional Yeast

Dinner: Miso-Glazed Salmon with Curried Chickpea and Spinach

Dessert: Chocolate Avocado Mousse

Day 18

Breakfast: Chia Pudding with Fruit

Snack: Bell Pepper Nachos

Lunch: BBQ-Pulled Chicken Sandwiches with Balsamic Glazed Carrots

Snack: Veggie Pinwheels

Dinner: Shrimp Scampi with Sweet Potato and Black Bean Hash

Dessert: Baked Cinnamon Apple Slices

Day 19

Breakfast: Greek Yogurt with Granola and Berries

Snack: Frozen Yogurt Bark

Lunch: Beef and Vegetable-Stir Fry with Lemon-Garlic Green Beans

Snack: Chocolate Banana Bites

Dinner: Shrimp and Spinach Stuffed Portobello Mushrooms with Garlic Mashed Cauliflower

Dessert: Coconut Rice Pudding

Day 20

Breakfast: Avocado and Egg Toast

Snack: Smoked Salmon and Cream Cheese Cucumber Bites

Lunch: Balsamic Glazed Chicken with Stovetop Ratatouille

Snack: Cheese and Crackers

Dinner: Teriyaki Glazed Salmon with Parmesan Roasted Broccoli

Dessert: Raspberry Lemon Sorbet

Day 21

Breakfast: Pineapple, Banana, and Spinach Smoothie

Snack: Spicy Roasted Chickpeas

Lunch: Sausage, Peppers, and Onions Skillets with Curried Chickpea and Spinach

Snack: Apple Slices with Almond Butter

Dinner: Seafood-Stuffed Bell Peppers with Oven-Roasted Root Vegetables

Dessert: Chocolate-Dipped Banana Bites

Day 22

Breakfast: Quinoa and Berry Breakfast Bowl

Snack: Greek Yogurt Ranch Dip with Veggies

Lunch: Rosemary Lemon Pork Chops with Cauliflower Fried Rice

Snack: Mini Caprese Skewers

Dinner: Lemon Garlic Shrimp and Asparagus with Sweet Potato and Black Bean Hash

Dessert: Mini Fruit Tarts

Day 23

Breakfast: Green Detox Smoothie

Snack: Celery Sticks with Cream Cheese and Everything Bagel Seasoning

Lunch: Moroccan-Spiced Beef Stew with Garlic-Roasted Brussels Sprouts

Snack: Avocado-Stuffed Cherry Tomatoes

Dinner: Pesto Baked Scallops with Sautéed Spinach with Garlic

Dessert: Lemon Blueberry Chia Pudding

Day 24

Breakfast: Veggie and Hummus Wrap

Snack: Cucumber Slices with Hummus

Lunch: Spinach and Feta Stuffed Chicken Breasts with Spicy Roasted Cauliflower

Snack: Ants on a Log

Dinner: Tilapia with Lemon Caper Sauce and Parmesan Roasted Broccoli

Dessert: Strawberry Banana Smoothie Bowl

Day 25

Breakfast: Cottage Cheese and Fruit Bowl

Snack: Easy Edamame

Lunch: Asian Turkey Lettuce Wraps with Balsamic Glazed Carrots

Snack: Peanut Butter and Chocolate Rice Cakes

Dinner: Spicy Orange Glazed Shrimp with Oven-Roasted Root Vegetables

Dessert: Mango Coconut Popsicles

Day 26

Breakfast: Multigrain Waffles with Fruit

Snack: Spinach and Artichoke Dip

Lunch: Eggplant Parmesan Stacks with Curried Chickpea and Spinach

Snack: Fruit Kabobs with Honey-Yogurt Drip

Dinner: Poached Cod with Tomato Salsa and Garlic Mashed Cauliflower

Dessert: Pineapple Coconut Macaroons

Day 27

Breakfast: Almond Butter and Apple Rice Cakes

Snack: Sliced Turkey and Cheese Roll-Ups

Lunch: Creamy Polenta with Roasted Vegetables and Lemon-Garlic Green Beans

Snack: Popcorn with Nutritional Yeast

Dinner: Lobster and Corn Chowder with Stovetop Ratatouille

Dessert: Almond Apricot Bites

Day 28

Breakfast: Spinach, Tomato, and Mozzarella Frittata

Snack: Bell Pepper Nachos

Lunch: Stuffed Portobello Mushrooms with Sweet and Sour Red Cabbage

Snack: Veggie Pinwheels

Dinner: Zucchini Fritters with Chickpea and Vegetable Curry

Dessert: Baked Cinnamon Apples

Day 29

Breakfast: Smoked Salmon and Avocado Rice Cake

Snack: Frozen Yogurt Bark

Lunch: Stuffed Bell Peppers with Garlic Mashed Cauliflower

Snack: Cheese and Crackers

Dinner: Seafood Paella with Lemon-Garlic Green Beans

Dessert: Fruit Kabobs with Honey Yogurt Dip

Day 30

Breakfast: Turkey Sausage and Veggie Scramble

Snack: Chocolate Banana Bites

Lunch: Chicken and Rice Stuffed Bell Peppers with Garlic-Roasted Brussels Sprouts

Snack: Greek Yogurt Ranch Dip with Veggies

Dinner: Miso-Glazed Salmon with Green Beans Almondine

Dessert: Dark Chocolate Bark with Dried Fruit and Nuts

CONCLUSION

This book serves as your ultimate guide to embracing a healthier lifestyle, with a primary focus on nurturing your heart health. By providing a customizable 30-day meal plan and a vast array of over 1500 delicious, low-sodium, and low-fat recipes, this cookbook aims to empower you to create a diverse and flavorful diet that does not compromise your heart health.

Starting a heart-healthy adventure can appear daunting initially, but this cookbook aims to facilitate a seamless and pleasurable shift. It offers a step-by-step approach to understanding the fundamentals of heart-healthy eating and equips you with the tools and knowledge necessary to create a sustainable and balanced diet. As you become more familiar with heart-healthy ingredients and cooking techniques, you'll start to experience the joy of creating nourishing and delicious meals for yourself and your loved ones.

A crucial element in sustaining a heart-friendly way of life involves embracing a comprehensive perspective on wellness. This includes making mindful, informed choices about the foods you consume and incorporating regular physical activity, stress management, and adequate sleep into your daily routine. Nurturing all aspects of your health will set the foundation for long-term success in preventing and managing heart disease.

Moreover, the heart-healthy cookbook emphasizes the importance of cultivating a positive mindset and attitude toward your health journey. This approach promotes engaging in the journey with eagerness, inquisitiveness, and kindness toward oneself, acknowledging that transformation requires time and that obstacles are an inherent aspect of development. Celebrating your progress and remaining open to learning and adaptation will create an empowering and supportive environment that fosters lasting change.

As you delve deeper into heart-healthy cooking and experiment with various recipes and ingredients, you'll likely notice a heart-healthy lifestyle's numerous benefits. Improved cardiovascular health is, of course, the primary goal, but you'll also experience increased energy levels, enhanced mental clarity, and better mood. By prioritizing your well-being, you're investing in your overall quality of life and setting the stage for a healthier and happier future.

Building a sense of community and having a support system is also crucial for maintaining a heart-healthy lifestyle. As you embark on your journey to better health, consider sharing your experiences, challenges, and successes with family and friends. By involving others in your health journey, you'll create a supportive network that can offer encouragement, advice, and motivation when needed. Moreover, your commitment to a heart-friendly lifestyle could motivate others to pursue their well-being, generating a chain reaction of beneficial transformations within your social circle.

As you venture into the world of heart-healthy cooking and embrace the journey to better health, remember to celebrate your achievements, remain open to growth, and share your experiences with others. In this way, you'll enhance your personal health while also encouraging the people around you to begin their individual journeys toward well-being. Here's to a lifetime of heart-healthy living and the many joys it brings!

INDEX

A

ALMOND APRICOT BITES, 98
ALMOND BUTTER AND APPLE RICE CAKES, 27
ANTS ON A LOG, 35
APPLE CINNAMON QUINOA BREAKFAST BOWL, 23
APPLE SLICES WITH ALMOND BUTTER, 33
ASIAN TURKEY LETTUCE WRAPS, 54
AVOCADO AND EGG TOAST, 30
AVOCADO AND TOMATO TOAST, 22
AVOCADO-STUFFED CHERRY TOMATOES, 34

B

BAKED CHICKEN FAJITA STUFFED PEPPERS, 41
BAKED CINNAMON APPLE SLICES, 93
BAKED CINNAMON APPLES, 98
BAKED COD WITH CHERRY TOMATOES AND OLIVES, 61
BAKED TILAPIA WITH MEDITERRANEAN SALSA, 59
BALSAMIC GLAZED CARROTS, 83
BALSAMIC GLAZED CHICKEN, 51
BALSAMIC-GLAZED PORK CHOPS, 43
BANANA OAT PANCAKES, 21
BBQ-PULLED CHICKEN SANDWICHES, 50
BEEF AND VEGETABLE STIR-FRY, 43
BEEF AND VEGETABLE-STIR FRY, 50
BEEF STIR-FRY WITH BROCCOLI, 41
BELL PEPPER NACHOS, 37
BERRY OATMEAL, 25
BUTTERNUT SQUASH AND APPLE SOUP, 74

C

CABBAGE AND POTATO SOUP, 80
CARROT AND GINGER SOUP, 81
CAULIFLOWER FRIED RICE, 83
CELERY STICKS WITH CREAM CHEESE AND EVERYTHING BAGEL SEASONING, 34
CHEESE AND CRACKERS, 39
CHIA PUDDING WITH FRUIT, 29
CHICKEN AND BROCCOLI STIR-FRY, 47
CHICKEN AND RICE STUFFED BELL PEPPERS, 45
CHICKEN AND VEGETABLE SOUP, 74
CHICKPEA AND VEGETABLE CURRY, 92
CHOCOLATE AVOCADO MOUSSE, 93
CHOCOLATE BANANA BITES, 38
CHOCOLATE-DIPPED BANANA BITES, 95
COCONUT RICE PUDDING, 94
COTTAGE CHEESE AND FRUIT BOWL, 26, 32
CRAB CAKES WITH LEMON AIOLI, 58
CREAMY CAULIFLOWER SOUP, 75
CREAMY MUSHROOM SOUP, 78
CREAMY POLENTA WITH ROASTED VEGETABLES, 90
CUCUMBER SLICES WITH HUMMUS, 35
CURRIED CHICKPEA AND SPINACH, 84

D

DARK CHOCOLATE BARK WITH DRIED FRUIT AND NUTS, 99

E

EASY CLAM SPAGHETTI, 59
EASY EDAMAME, 35

EASY FRUIT SALAD, 93
EGGPLANT PARMESAN STACKS, 89

F

FROZEN YOGURT BARK, 38
FRUIT KABOBS WITH HONEY YOGURT DIP, 99
FRUIT KABOBS WITH HONEY-YOGURT DRIP, 36

G

GARLIC BUTTER SCALLOPS, 62
GARLIC HERB PORK TENDERLOIN, 46
GARLIC MASHED CAULIFLOWER, 87
GARLIC-ROASTED BRUSSELS SPROUTS, 83
GREEK CHICKEN PITA POCKETS, 49
GREEK YOGURT AND BERRY PARFAIT, 24
GREEK YOGURT RANCH DIP WITH VEGGIES, 33
GREEK YOGURT WITH GRANOLA AND BERRIES, 29
GREEK-STYLE GRILLED CHICKEN, 42
GREEN BEANS ALMONDINE, 87
GREEN DETOX SMOOTHIE, 31
GRILLED PORTOBELLO MUSHROOM BURGERS, 48

H

HEARTY VEGETABLE AND BARLEY SOUP, 77

L

LEMON BLUEBERRY CHIA PUDDING, 96
LEMON GARLIC BAKED COD, 56
LEMON GARLIC BAKED TILAPIA, 65
LEMON GARLIC SHRIMP AND ASPARAGUS, 67
LEMON-GARLIC GEREN BEANS, 85

LOBSTER AND CORN CHOWDER, 70

M

MANGO COCONUT POPSICLES, 97
MINESTRONE SOUP, 75
MINI CAPRESE SKEWERS, 34
MINI FRUIT TARTS, 95
MISO VEGETABLE SOUP, 80
MISO-GLAZED SALMON, 64
MOROCCAN-SPICED BEEF STEW, 53
MULTIGRAIN WAFFLES WITH FRUIT, 27
MUSHROOM BARLEY SOUP, 73

O

ONE-PAN SHRIMP AND ASPARAGUS, 58
OVEN-ROASTED ROOT VEGETABLE, 89
OVERNIGHT CHIA PUDDING, 22

P

PAN-SEARED SCALLOPS WITH GARLIC SPINACH, 57
PARMESAN ROASTED BROCCOLI, 87
PEA AND MINT SOUP, 81
PEANUT BUTTER AND BANANA SMOOTHIE, 24
PEANUT BUTTER AND CHOCOLATE RICE CAKES, 36
PESTO BAKED SCALLOPS, 68
PHILLY CHEESESTEAK STUFFED PEPPERS, 49
PINEAPPLE COCONUT MACAROONS, 97
PINEAPPLE, BANANA, AND SPINACH SMOOTHIE, 30
POACHED COD WITH TOMATO SALSA, 69
POPCORN WITH NUTRITIONAL YEAST, 37
PORK TENDERLOIN WITH BALSAMIC GLAZE, 40

POTATO AND LEEK SOUP, 81
POTATO LEEK SOUP, 76

Q

QUINOA AND BERRY BREAKFAST BOWL, 30

R

RASPBERRY LEMON SORBET, 94
ROASTED RED PEPPER AND TOMATO SOUP, 76

S

SALMON WITH DILL YOGURT SAUCE, 57
SAUTÉED SPINACH WITH GARLIC, 88
SEAFOOD PAELLA, 61
SEAFOOD-STUFFED BELL PEPPERS, 66
SEARED AHI TUNA WITH MANGO SALSA, 60
SHEET PAN SAUSAGE AND VEGETABLES, 44
SHRIMP AND SPINACH STUFFED PORTOBELLO MUSHROOMS, 65
SHRIMP AND VEGGIE STIR-FRY, 56
SHRIMP SCAMPI, 64
SLICED TURKEY AND CHEESE ROLL-UPS, 37
SLOW COOKER BEEF STEW, 44
SMOKED SALMON AND AVOCADO RICE CAKE, 28
SMOKED SALMON AND CREAM CHEESE CUCUMBER BITES, 39
SPAGHETTI SQUASH BOLOGNESE, 45
SPICED LENTIL SOUP, 73
SPICED RED LENTIL SOUP, 79
SPICY ORANGE GLAZED SHRIMP, 69
SPICY ROASTED CAULIFLOWER, 86
SPICY ROASTED CHICKPEAS, 33
SPINACH AND ARTICHOKE DIP, 36
SPINACH AND FETA STUFFED CHICKEN BREASTS, 54
SPINACH AND MUSHROOM EGG WHITE SCRAMBLE, 21
SPINACH AND WHITE BEAN SOUP, 72
SPINACH, TOMATO, AND MOZZARELLA FRITTATA, 27
STOVETOP RATATOUILLE, 86
STRAWBERRY BANANA SMOOTHIE BOWL, 96
STUFFED BELL PEPPERS, 84
STUFFED PORTOBELLO MUSHROOMS, 91
SWEET AND SOUR RED CABBAGE, 88
SWEET POTATO AND BLACK BEAN HASH, 85

T

TERIYAKI GLAZED SALMOND, 66
TILAPIA WITH LEMON CAPER SAUCE, 68
TOMATO BASIL SOUP, 72
TROPICAL GREEN SMOOTHIE, 26
TURKEY MEATBALL SUBS, 47
TURKEY MEATBALLS, 40
TURKEY SAUSAGE AND VEGGIE SCRAMBLE, 28

V

VEGETABLE OMELET, 25
VEGGIE AND EGG BREAKFAST BURRITO, 23
VEGGIE AND HUMMUS WRAP, 31
VEGGIE PINWHEELS, 38

W

WHITE BEAN AND KALE SOUP, 78

Z

ZUCCHINI AND CORN CHOWDER, 79
ZUCCHINI FRITTERS, 91

Made in the USA
Monee, IL
30 December 2023

50799716R00070